The Boy and His Death

Marga Beukeboom

iUniverse, Inc.
New York   Bloomington

The Boy and His Death

iUniverse books may be ordered through booksellers or by contacting:

iUniverse
1663 Liberty Drive
Bloomington, IN 47403
www.iuniverse.com
1-800-Authors (1-800-288-4677)

ISBN: 978-1-4502-2841-1 (sc)
ISBN: 978-1-4502-2843-5 (dj)
ISBN: 978-1-4502-2842-8 (ebk)

Printed in the United States of America

iUniverse rev. date: 6/3/2010

For Zoë

A memorial to my son, Benjamin,
who battled his disease in a unique and spiritual way.

Contents

Introduction

This is the true story of my son Benjamin, who battled testicular cancer for three years and died from the disease at the age of twenty-four. Even though testicular cancer is among the most treatable cancers, and, according to the American Cancer Society[1], 95 percent of patients with the condition beat it and survive at least five years, that still leaves 5 percent who don't. Men do die of this disease. And most of them are young, like Benjamin, in the prime of their lives.

I am writing this book so that not only young men but also their parents become aware of the seriousness and dangers of this awful disease—to make them aware that even young men can die from testicular cancer. A study done at the University of Huddersfield in England, which appeared in the *European Journal of Cancer Care*[2], showed that most young men still don't know much about the signs, symptoms, or risks of this cancer. I did not know anything about testicular cancer, had not even heard of it, until my son was diagnosed with this disease. Testicular cancer is the most common cancer affecting young men between twenty and thirty-four years old. More than half of all testicular cancers occur in men under thirty-five years old, while only 15 percent of testicular cancers are diagnosed in men over fifty.

---

1.   American Cancer Society, "Detailed Guide: Testicular Cancer," American Cancer Society, www.cancer.org/docroot/CRI/content/CRI_2_4_1X_What_are_ the_key_statistics_for_testicular_cancer_41.asp?sitearea=.

2.   Moore and Annie Topping, "Young Men's Knowledge of Testicular Cancer and Testicular Self-examination: A Lost Opportunity?" *European Journal of Cancer Care,* 8 (2001): 137–142, www3.interscience.wiley.com/journal/119096075/ abstract.

Conventional treatment[3] (chemotherapy) for testicular cancer is very effective, and the vast majority of patients are cured.

Researchers from Cancer Care Ontario and the U.S. Centers for Disease Control and Prevention presented evidence, published in the January 26, 1999, issue of the *Canadian Medical Association Journal,* that the number of men diagnosed with testicular cancer—men primarily in their twenties and thirties—has increased almost 60 percent over the past three decades, one of the steepest climbs for any known form of cancer.

Testicular cancer is still quite rare, striking only about 8,400 men a year in the United States[4]. Of that number, 380 men are expected to die of the disease each year, which in my opinion is 380 too many. In the United Kingdom, 2,100 men are diagnosed with testicular cancer every year[5]—eight men every working day. With this book, I hope to not only tell my son's story but to increase awareness of testicular cancer among young people. If warning signs are ignored, testicular cancer may spread to the lymph nodes, lungs, and brain. Advanced cancer is more difficult to treat successfully and may lead to death. Males age fifteen and older should examine themselves regularly and continue the process through their thirties. Self-examination is particularly important because cancer of the testes is usually asymptomatic. That means there are no symptoms, such as stomach aches, fever, or pain, which might clue young men in to a potential medical problem.

There are, however, warning signs:

- One testicle may swell or feel abnormally heavy.
- Male breasts may enlarge and feel tender.
- A sore may develop which does not heal.
- A small, painless lump may develop on a testicle.

Instructions for how to perform a TSE (testicular self-examination) can be found on the Internet at several sites, including:

http://tcrc.acor.org/tcexam.html

---

3.   *Wikipedia, The Free Encyclopedia,* "Testicular Cancer," http://en.wikipedia.org/wiki/Testicular_cancer (accessed 2009); National Cancer Institute, "Testicular Cancer," National Cancer Institute, www.cancer.gov/cancertopics/types/testicular.

4.   National Cancer Institute, "Testicular Cancer," National Cancer Institute, www.cancer.gov/cancertopics/types/testicular/.

5.   Cancer Research UK, "Testicular Cancer Statistics and Outlook," Cancer Research UK, www.cancerhelp.org.uk/type/testicular-cancer/treatment/testicular-cancer-statistics-and-outlook.

www.cancerhelp.org.uk/help/default.asp?page=3570
www.nlm.nih.gov/medlineplus/ency/article/003909.htm

Nowadays there are even YouTube movies on the Web teaching men how to perform self-exams.

There are several success stories from people, such as Lance Armstrong, Tom Green, and other celebrities, who did beat this disease. There are also several books describing the success of their battle. However, we hardly hear the other side—testicular cancer is still a killer. There are no testicular cancer books in which the story does not have a happy ending, as far as I know. This book has no such happy ending. I hope to show young men and their parents, friends, and relatives that if help is not sought immediately, the battle that lay ahead can end in death. Waiting can be fatal. The battle Benjamin went through—the pain, the agony, the emotional roller coaster, the nightmare of this disease called cancer—is almost indescribable. Fighting testicular cancer will control your life day and night.

I have learned through this battle that when the cancer has spread, conventional medicine does not know all the answers and cannot guarantee survival. As you will read in the following chapters, Benjamin experimented with several alternative treatments. Some were somewhat successful, just like chemotherapy was somewhat successful. But the alternative treatments could not guarantee survival either. Through the three years that Benjamin was fighting the battle, I researched everything I could find about both conventional therapies and alternative therapies. Before Benjamin was diagnosed, I never had looked into alternative therapies, or into conventional treatments, for that matter. In the beginning I was simply shocked when Benjamin told me that he wanted to try alternative therapies first. Like so many of us, I was ignorant of all those therapies and felt it was all quackery, until I started looking into the various available alternatives and read all the testimonials from people for whom alternative therapies had worked. I started reading anything I could find on the Internet and searched any alternative books I saw in bookstores.

I am convinced to this day that if Benjamin had followed the alternative protocols that were suggested to him, and if he had had the testicle removed in the beginning, he would have had a better chance of surviving. He would not have had to go through the chemotherapies.

His alternative therapy of Laetrile[6] was effective, in the sense that it brought down his tumor markers and stabilized the cancer. However, oncologists refused to acknowledge its effectiveness, even though his tumor markers reduced dramatically while he was on Laetrile. Their mind-set was much too focused on the traditional therapies, such as chemo. While Benjamin was on Laetrile, nobody paid any attention to detoxifying his body, which is important to get rid of the dead cancer cells. At the time I did not know enough about detoxifying the body or its importance. However, rather than condemning one approach to fighting cancer over another, my sincerest wish is that both the conventional medical world and the alternative world may someday work more closely together to find answers to finally cure cancer.

Benjamin, this book is dedicated to you. I love you. It was a great honor to be your mother. I am proud of you, and one day we will meet again. For now you are in my heart every single day for the rest of my life.

---

6.   Laetrile, also known as amygdalin or vitamin B-17, is a nitriloside found in many foods, including seeds from apricots, peaches, and apples, and in millet, buckwheat, and many other grains.

CHAPTER 1

A Celebration of Benjamin's Life

Benjamin Hyman

2-2-1978   12-02-2002[7]

This is just the beginning ...

Today, Saturday, February 16, 2002, my son Benjamin was buried. Zoë, my daughter; Frido, her partner at the time; my husband Mike and I got up early. We had to go to the funeral home to prepare and to make sure everything was set up and ready to go before the first people arrived to express their condolences and to say good-bye to Benjamin. It was another beautiful day, nothing but sunshine, just like the previous four days. The sky was totally blue, not a cloud to be seen. Strange, I thought, that all of the week before until Tuesday it had been terrible weather. Rain had poured down, with no end in sight. On the morning of February 12, the sky broke, and the sun had not stopped shining since. It was as if Benjamin had purposely chosen that day to die, the

---

7.   The European date format is day, month, and year. February 12, 2002, was the date of Benjamin's passing.

1

day the Chinese New Year started, as if he were aware that the weather would change from totally miserable to perfect.

Since Tuesday we had been busy getting the funeral arranged. The past four days had been very hectic. Relatives and friends had been dropping by, expressing their sorrow and condolences. We had been so busy preparing for the funeral that we had not had a chance to fully realize that my son Benjamin had passed. Maybe it was better that way. We had been busy designing Benjamin's mourning card and making arrangements for the funeral. The day he died, the funeral home people had come by to pick up his body and to explain the issues that needed to be taken care of. They had shown us their collection of cards and the different layouts that they printed and arranged. In the Netherlands it is custom to send *mourn cards* to relatives and friends to announce the passing of a beloved one. At the same time the card serves to let people know when the funeral will take place and at what time and day they can say good-bye. But the cards the funeral home offered all looked like cards for old people, not for a young man of only twenty-four. They did not fit Benjamin; they would not represent Benjamin the right way. For that reason, we decided to design our own.

Zoë, Frido, Mike, and I were all computer literate and familiar with various software packages, including graphic programs. We had to hurry, though. The card needed to be designed, printed, and made ready for mailing by Wednesday evening, because the funeral was scheduled for Saturday. We decided to put Benjamin's photo on the card. I found a passport picture of Benjamin in one of the cabinet draws in his bedroom. It was the same picture he had used for his driving license. It was beautiful—he looked at his best in this picture. It had been taken the year before, in April, when he had to take his driving test in the Netherlands, where his Texas driver's license was not valid. Mike remembered when Benjamin went to the photographer to have the picture taken. He had his photo taken three times, as he had not been satisfied with the results. Mike had jokingly said, "Benjamin, who cares? The photo is just for your diver's license." I was now very grateful that Benjamin had been so vain. We used this portrait for his mourn card. Frido and Zoë went to the local photo shop to have it enlarged. It came out unexpectedly good, considering it was just a small passport picture. Before I placed the enlarged photo in a beautiful frame that

Zoë had purchased at the photo store, Frido scanned in the photo and started on Mike's Macintosh to see what he could do to design the card. I then placed the photo in the frame and found a perfect spot for it in the shelved wall unit in the living room, overlooking all of us.

Zoë and I started looking at text that would be appropriate to add to the card. We went through the examples the funeral home had left behind. Normally, these cards started with some kind of religious phrase or rhyme. Benjamin was not raised in any religion. His father is of Jewish descent, and I was raised a Catholic. Both Benjamin and Zoë did spend their first couple of school years at a Protestant school and were raised in a somewhat Christian environment. However, we did not feel that a religious phrase would be justified. Mike suggested we used a couple of lines from Robert Frost's poem "The Road Not Taken." I found that the lines from the poem were extremely fitting because when he was first diagnosed with cancer Benjamin had made choices that were not the norm. We decided to put a couple of the phrases on the card, below his picture, which was on the left side of the card when you opened it. On the right side the text was going to be printed. Simple text, just informing recipients that Benjamin had passed, when the funeral was going take place, and where people could go to express their condolences and say good-bye to Benjamin. The card itself was going to be purple. Once we had the design of the card behind us, we needed to have it printed at a local printer. Frido and Mike went down and were guaranteed it would be ready the next day.

It was not until ten or eleven o'clock when friends and family left that night. After a very hectic and emotional day, Mike and I finally sat down to rest a bit before going to bed. I looked at my beautiful son's picture, the picture we had just enlarged, now displayed on the shelf in the wall unit. Benjamin winked at me. What I saw was real. Benjamin winked at me. "He winked at me, Mike!" I shouted. "He just winked at me!" It gave me such a burst of energy, and very happy feelings spread all over. Was I imagining this? Or was it a sign to show me he was okay and that I did not need to worry?

The next day, once the cards had been picked up, we gathered all the addresses of friends, family, and relatives. As a team we addressed the envelopes, inserted the cards, and stamped the envelopes. I took all the envelopes to the post office and was guaranteed that the mourn cards would be delivered within the Netherlands overnight. The next step was to arrange the service. A couple of days before Benjamin died, I had asked him if he wanted a formal service, but because he was not raised in any religion he said he did not think so. Instead, as a family, we thought it would be nice if we could present a photo slideshow of his life, and several people could then speak a few words in memory of Benjamin. We selected random pictures from babyhood until his adult life. Mike scanned all the pictures into the computer and created a continuous slideshow. Then we needed to decide what music we were going to play during the service. Benjamin had one big hero, the song writer and musician Prince, so we looked at all his Prince CDs and decided on three songs. We also decided to play some of the music Benjamin had mixed himself and recorded on his computer. We burned a CD with the songs to be played during the service. Both the music and the speeches needed to be timed, as altogether forty-five minutes were allocated for the service before the funeral itself.

Everything seemed to fit perfectly and fell into place. It was like Benjamin was guiding us, helping us picking the songs. On the day before the funeral everything was ready. Frido and Zoë picked up a beamer and rented a large screen. I had been busy typing up the few words I wanted to say during the service in a large, easily readable font, which I printed out. I read the text out loud about fifty times. Every time I read certain paragraphs I had to cry. I told myself: "You cannot cry at the funeral." I was not allowed to cry; I needed to be strong so that people would be able to follow me. I had to get it right. So I kept reading the text over and over until I finally managed to do so without crying. Zoë decided she would recite Robert Frost's poem, and Wayne, Benjamin's father, would read an e-mail his sister Susan had sent that she asked Wayne to read, as she herself was unable to come over from the United States to attend the funeral.

We arrived at the funeral home Saturday morning and walked into the service room where the coffin with Benjamin's body was. Tons of flowers and bouquets had been arranged on the floor around the coffin. Flowers came from people who were not able to attend the funeral but also from friends and relatives who would be attending. As fast as we could, we put the screen, computer, and beamer in place. We tested the stereo equipment that was available from the funeral home; we tested the microphone and the slide show. Everything was in order. Downstairs there was a large gathering room, where we would first welcome those who came to say good-bye to Benjamin and express their condolences. We had two registers for people to sign. We—Mike, Zoë, Frido, Wayne, and myself—all stood there, waiting for the first people to arrive. The first person who came to express condolences was Benjamin's first serious girlfriend, the girlfriend he fell in love with when he was only seventeen. He kept in touch with her even after he left Holland and they had officially broken up.

Soon the assembly room was filled with friends, relatives, and neighbors. All had come to say good-bye. We welcomed them with a cup of coffee and apple pie, Benjamin's favorite. After a while, we all went upstairs to the room where Benjamin's body lay in state. The room looked like a chapel room, like a church. Music was playing softly as we entered. People sat down. Prince's "Let's Go Crazy" started playing, loud and clear. It was a fitting beginning to this celebration—Benjamin's celebration of his life.

"Let's Go Crazy" finished playing. It was then time for me to address the family, friends, and relatives who had come to say good-bye to Benjamin. I walked up onto the podium and stood behind the microphone. Before I spoke the few words about Benjamin that I had prepared, I first mentioned that the song they just heard was from Prince, Benjamin's hero. Then I started my speech.

Benjamin, my son ...

Benjamin died at home, very much at peace with himself. Mike and I were with him when he died. He knew his time had come, and he accepted it. Benjamin was definitely not afraid to die. Since the beginning of this year, Benjamin's health had deteriorated very rapidly, and before we realized it Benjamin was once again a very sick young man. The past couple of weeks I took care of Benjamin at home, and that allowed me the time to accept and to have peace with knowing that he would leave us soon.

I am proud of my son; I admire him and salute him. Not once did he complain during the past three years; not once did he ask, "Why?

Why me?" He had so much pain; he suffered so much. Yet he bore it with courage. We can all learn from him. We are sad for our own selfish reasons. But Benjamin would like all of us to have peace with it and accept his death.

Today we celebrate his life. Do not mourn his death …

Benjamin's earthly life started at the Rembrandt van Rijnstraat in Bunschoten, the Netherlands. Benjamin was a very pleasant little boy, a bit shy maybe, a good-looking little blond guy. From early on in his life he had a special friend: Klaas. Klaas, with whom he grew up, was a friend who remained true to Benjamin through the years until his last days here on earth. They couldn't have been older than three years when they became buddies. Benjamin attended the nursery school D'Arke, which was located in our street. However, Benjamin never really enjoyed nursery school very much. Even then he was already ahead of his time. He felt nursery school was too childish for him. One day he even decided to run away from school—a little secret Benjamin just recently shared with his youngest five-year-old sister Sarah[8]. The result was that Sarah, together with one of her girlfriends, also decided to run away from school. His elementary years were spent at the Nieuw Baarnse School. He joined soccer when he was six years old, playing and training at the Baarnse Soccer Club. The six elementary school years were no problem for Benjamin—he performed splendidly.

We already knew Benjamin was a very intelligent young man. A cito test[9] result of 550 out of 550 proved it. We, his parents, would have preferred that Benjamin had attended the Baarns Lyceum for his higher education. Benjamin himself preferred to go to the Griftland College, where both his sister Zoë and his friend Klaas were following their educations. There was a lot of partying, a little studying during those years. Whenever I asked, "Benjamin, did you complete your homework?" the answer was always, "As good as …" I knew very well he had not even opened his school books. After his high school years,

---

8.   Benjamin shared this "secret" with his then five-year-old sister in autumn 2001.

9.   Cito tests are end of elementary school tests, exams that are annually administered to approx. 160,000 final-year elementary school pupils in the Netherlands.

Benjamin had a go just for a year at the Midland College in Amersfoort. One day he just told the teachers he was leaving and going to the United States. Together he and his stepbrother Kenneth had their first go at living by themselves in their own apartment. They studied and worked in Austin, Texas, learning to stand on their own two feet. Beginning the summer 1997, Benjamin met Sifu, a wise Chinese Tai Chi teacher. Benjamin took up Tai Chi lessons; to be able to pay for his lessons he helped his Chinese teacher in his herbal shop. Since that time, Benjamin became very much interested in herbs and natural medicines. Thanks to this wise Chinese teacher, Benjamin also learned a lot about himself.

During the summer of 1998 it became obvious there was something wrong,[10] without knowing exactly what was wrong. During the summer Benjamin returned to the Netherlands, looking for answers, looking to find himself. Feeling somewhat better, Benjamin decided at the end of 1998 to once again continue with studies in the United States. Beginning in January 1999, he became very enthusiastic about his education. During March of that year he found a new apartment and lived by himself. Self-assured, proud, and full of confidence, he showed his new home to his sister Zoë and me in April when we went over for a short visit from the Netherlands. During that visit Benjamin very carefully told me he was afraid there was something wrong. In May 1999, he was diagnosed with cancer. When Benjamin informed me about the diagnosis, he asked me to respect and to support his decisions. One of his remarks was: "If I survive this, then that is reason to celebrate. If I do not survive, then it still will be a reason to celebrate." Today we are here to celebrate his life, his illusion, his death ...

Now I would like to read a couple of paragraphs from a story Benjamin wrote[11]. He wrote this in December 1998, when he was twenty years old, before he knew he had cancer. The story is called "The Boy and His Death."

---

10.   In the summer of 1998 Benjamin began having sweating problems, which made him feel embarrassed and somewhat depressed. Breaking up with a girlfriend at this time did not help the situation. Excessive sweating can sometimes be a sign of serious underlying conditions, and looking back, I believe this excessive sweating was an early sign of cancer.

11.   The complete story can be found at the end of this book in the Afterword.

He was only twenty-four when they met. Death stood there, facing him. What used to make up his surroundings had disappeared. The boy examined Death closely and noticed the kind expression on his face. The boy must have looked puzzled when Death asked him what he wished to have answered. "I don't know where to start," the boy said. "There is so much I wish to know." Suddenly he realized the past twenty-four years were merely a creation of his imagination, which took place in a fraction of a moment. Those years never existed! In fact the whole concept of time started to lose its meaning. "At some point you will forget that it is all your imagination," Death had told him. Like magic Death appeared before him. "But those years on earth were real! How can reality and imagination be so similar?" the boy asked. "That's because they are the same. They only differ in meaning, which we add to them."

The boy could see clearly what the illusion held. Hey, he had lived it for twenty-four illusionary years. Over and over again. "What about my mother, my sister? Were they real?" the boy asked Death. "Real in a sense you all shared the same illusion. In the illusion of your mother, you are her son. In your sister's illusion, you play the part of brother. Collective dreaming, I like to call it." (We all wake up sooner or later.) "But now that I have woken up from my dream, what happens to my part in the illusions/dreams of the people close to me? Will I still exist to them?" "This is difficult to explain but easy to understand. To them you disappeared out of what they call their life. They don't have a clue of where you went. They don't know you simply 'woke up.' In your case you woke up during their lives. So you weren't responding to their illusion of you anymore. To them you are dead. Just like your grandfather was to you." The boy started to look back at his illusion. His birth, his years growing up to be a child, his school years, finally his last years before he died of cancer. He understood that it was all part of his own imagination, and he recognized the blessing of his illness. It had enabled him to wake up to a place where he was the creator, a place where time had no meaning at all. A place without boundaries and limitations. A place where one and zero were the same. A place where his body had no beginning and no end. A place so magnificently free of everything. The boy tried to think of an ending to his story. No matter how hard he tried, the right words to end the story wouldn't appear. Suddenly he realized there was no ending to this story. This was only the beginning …

I finished my speech with a poem Benjamin had written at the same time he had written his story.

Dedicated to my only friend
He who will be there for me in the end
He who will take my pain away
On my final day
He who I can always count on
Even after I am gone.
Death …

I stepped down and returned to my seat. The next Prince song played: "I Wish You Heaven." Zoë stood up and recited Robert Frost's poem "The Road Not Taken," the poem that fitted Benjamin so well.

Two roads diverged in a yellow wood,
And sorry I could not travel both
And be one traveler, long I stood
And looked down one as far as I could
To where it bent in the undergrowth;

Then took the other, as just as fair,
And having perhaps the better claim
Because it was grassy and wanted wear;
Though as for that the passing there
Had worn them really about the same,

And both that morning equally lay
In leaves no step had trodden black.
Oh, I kept the first for another day!
Yet knowing how way leads on to way,
I doubted if I should ever come back.

> I shall be telling this with a sigh
> Somewhere ages and ages hence:
> Two roads diverged in a wood, and I—
> I took the one less traveled by,
> And that has made all the difference.

Another song was played, and Benjamin's father read the e-mail he had received from his sister Susan: Susan, who had become very dear to me and who had become an important supportive person through the entire ordeal of this nightmare, this battle called cancer that not just Benjamin but all of us had fought. Susan, who lives in the United States, could not make it to the funeral, but had e-mailed to ask if Wayne, her brother, would have the strength to read out loud some words she had written:

> Dear Wayne, Marga, Zoë, Mike, family, and friends,
>
> Sadly I could not make the trip to speak these words in person … to share with all of you of how my nephew Benjamin not only touched my life but touched my heart … He was a free spirit … who sought answers to the most complex questions … always curious … always searching
>
> His contagious smile … his quizzical mind … his infinite search to discover the "Why?" no matter what the topic … His love of nature and always seeking the beauty within— never content with the book cover but more interested in the content … His intellect and passion for the mysterious … he was a complex young man … who many may not have understood, but that was all part of the unique package we knew and loved as Benjamin … I didn't have the pleasure as many of you did of watching him grow up into a handsome free spirited man … but I did have the joy of spending some quality time with him a couple of years ago. And each minute we shared together was always more interesting, more fun—more poignant than the last … we talked, we teased, we laughed, we even agreed to disagree, many times I may add. But we always understood and respected each other—we would do this many times—sometimes as we shared french fries … he loved french fries and apple pie.

Benjamin was a very brave young man ... he lived and died on his terms, in his own way ... with those that loved him the most close by his side ... as he crossed over to the other side. Now where he is whole, healthy and looking over those that he loved—his Mom, Dad, sister, family, and friends ...

My very last words to him were "I love you, Benjamin" ... and in his weak voice, he replied "I love you" ... I knew then it would be the last time I would ever hear his voice ... I am sad ... for me ... But I'm at peace because I know he is no longer in pain ... His spirit lives on ... his memory will remain forever in my heart and in my mind, as it will in all those that had the joy of knowing and loving Benjamin ...

Celebrate his life ... because he would have it no other way ... I will miss you ... but you are never far away—I can feel your presence in everything beautiful ...

Benjamin means son ... son of my right hand ... He is your son ... he is our son ... he is unforgettable ...
I love you, Benjamin ...

Susan

It was hard for Wayne to read those beautiful words out loud without becoming emotional. The music Benjamin himself had mixed started to play. The music started with words spoken by a man, who sounded Indian. The words were about the different religions, the different beliefs, and the necessity that we all come together, to respect all nations, all religions. Regretfully, the words were not that clear, and I am not sure if everyone at the service did understand. I don't have any idea where Benjamin got those wise words from. Benjamin's mix sounded beautiful, perfect.

Next it was Klaas' turn to say a few words. I knew it took a lot of courage for him to do so. He had expressed concerns about speaking before a large audience, if you will. But, together with Mariska, he stepped forward, and Klaas quoted a few words from the conversation Benjamin and Klaas had had only two days before Benjamin died.

"Benjamin, we spoke about life when you said: 'That is easy for you to talk about ...' We spoke about death when you said: 'Now, that's easy for me to talk about.' You have always lived. There is no death. Just a temporarily farewell, but even that is an illusion. Dear Benjamin, the sun rises at the same point as it goes under. Just like the sun that never really goes under, there will never be an end to the journey of our souls. We love you, you are our best friend, we will miss you."

Once the service was over, people were given one last chance to walk past the coffin and say good-bye to my beautiful, courageous son. Then the coffin was closed. The caretakers took the coffin and placed it in the hearse. We all walked silently behind the hearse from the funeral home to the cemetery. Benjamin had wanted the funeral to take place with respect and dignity. Walking behind the hearse to the cemetery was definitely respectful and dignifying. It was a short walk, maybe ten minutes. The cemetery in Baarn where Benjamin is buried is beautiful. The entrance is magnificent, with beautiful arches in front of the building, which lead up to the large cemetery. The parklike cemetery has very large trees, and the graves are gracefully arranged below and between the trees. Especially in summer, it feels like you are walking in a forest. I wished Benjamin could have seen it himself before he died. When it became clear that he was not going to survive this awful disease, I had asked Benjamin where he would want to be buried. He did not know, and therefore I suggested Baarn, as that was the place where he was born. Benjamin agreed. Now we were there, his last resting place, full of tall trees, beautiful bushes—well maintained and very peaceful.

The coffin was taken out of the hearse. Flowers lay on top of the coffin. Mike, Ken, Klaas, and other family members carried the coffin to his grave. We all gathered around the grave, and Klaas' father spoke the last words. He mentioned how Benjamin had grown up together with his son Klaas, how Benjamin had been like a son to him, how Benjamin had been like a brother to Klaas' younger brother. That he never had said "I love you" to Benjamin and that he felt he needed to say it now. Because he sincerely loved Benjamin in his own special way, just as his wife and kids loved Benjamin. He said he loved his children, something he did not tell them that often. Now he realized how important those words were, not just then during the burial but every day. In silence we all walked back from the cemetery to the funeral home. There we thanked everybody for their support and sympathy. Benjamin's life on earth was no longer.

This was just the beginning …

CHAPTER 2

The News

Two roads diverged in a yellow wood,
And sorry I could not travel both
And be one traveler, long I stood
And looked down one as far as I could …

Two roads diverged in a wood, and I—
I took the one less traveled by,
And that has made all the difference.

From: "The Road Not Taken," by Robert Frost

During the early months of 1999 I temporarily resided in Rotterdam, the Netherlands, for my job as a Systems Application and Products (SAP) data processing consultant[12], away from my husband Mike and my son Benjamin. There I was, back in my country of birth, the country

---

12.   SAP is a German company that is the market and technology leader in business management software. As a functional consultant, I was responsible for evaluating the demands of the client for what the system software should be able to do. I translated their demands in the business processes and made sure that the new

I had lived in for almost my entire life. Then I met Mike, my second husband, in the mid-eighties while he was stationed in the Netherlands. Mike is an American. In the early 1990s, Mike and I moved from the Netherlands to Austin, Texas. My daughter Zoë and my son Benjamin joined us a couple of years later. Before joining us in the States, they lived with their dad in the Netherlands. Zoë lived in the United States for just over a year before she returned to the Netherlands, where she is still living today. Benjamin had temporarily gone back to the Netherlands in 1998 to try to find out what was wrong with him and why he was suffering from excessive sweating, which embarrassed him and had taken away his self-confidence and his self-assurance. But by 1998 he was back in Austin. He returned just before Christmas, after having lived in Holland for seven months.

During March, while I worked in Rotterdam, I received a couple of long e-mails from Benjamin. In contrast to the previous year, Benjamin was once again full of hope, full of enthusiasm, feeling good about himself and his future. In January he had started school again, attending Austin Community College. And he had just found an apartment and had signed the lease. He e-mailed me that he could move in any time, even though the lease did not take effect until April 1. He was pleased with the allowance he received from me for his studies. Benjamin figured that by working fifteen to twenty hours a week he would be able to supplement his income and take care of his studies and his responsibilities. He explained to me how thrilled he was with the apartment, what a beautiful area it was, full of tall trees and very close to the center of Austin. Everything was within walking distance, or only a bike ride away. "You should come to Austin soon," he e-mailed me, "to see the apartment. It is a super location," he wrote. "The entire neighborhood is full of green tall trees." Benjamin greatly respected anything to do with nature, with Mother Earth. Zilker Park was only a three-minute bike ride away. Lake Austin Boulevard was only a two-minute walk. He was proud that things went well at school. His English essay had been accepted, no "rewrite" or "revise." He had received a high grade for math. He said how much fun it was to go to school, now that he realized why he was going to school. He was pleased that spring

---

system software to be implemented reacted in a manner according to the client's requirements.

break was over, glad to get back to his studies. It was nice to receive these positive e-mails, and I replied that I was happy for him. I was so happy that everything was going well, that his future looked bright. I had not seen him this happy for a long time. I e-mailed Benjamin that I would try to come and visit soon.

In the third week in April, Zoë and I flew to Austin. My company allowed me to fly back to Texas frequently. I decided to take Zoë along to see her brother, as she had not seen him since he had returned to Texas the Christmas before. The purpose for the visit to Austin was twofold. Of course we came for Benjamin, wanting to share his joy and happiness and to see his new home. But we also visited because of Mike, as it was his birthday on April 24. Mike had been by himself since the beginning of February when I accepted the project assignment in Rotterdam.

It was nice to be home again, even though it was only for a week. Benjamin proudly showed his apartment to Zoë and me. We celebrated Mike's birthday. We went shopping and enjoyed our short break. Then one evening when I was already in bed, the phone rang. It was Benjamin. He was calling from the police station. The police had stopped and arrested him, as he had an outstanding traffic ticket. I was aware of this custom in Texas; if you had not paid a traffic ticket, the police would lock you up. In Holland that was unthinkable. There they would just send you a reminder to pay. I told Benjamin not to worry and said I would come down to the police station to pay the outstanding fee, and he would be released. While I was getting dressed, Benjamin called again and told me that I better bring a lawyer with me, because it wasn't as simple as just paying the ticket to get him out of jail. Apparently the police had searched his car and had found a butterfly knife in the back of his car.

Bring a lawyer? Where would I get a lawyer from at this time at night? I never before had needed a lawyer.

Mike got up as well, and together we looked through the Yellow Pages to find a lawyer. We picked one who was close to the center of Austin and to the police station. Mike rang this lawyer, and he promised to come down to the city jail within half an hour. Mike and I left to go to the city jail to get Benjamin out. We paid the lawyer his fee, and he went to see Benjamin after discussing the matter with the officials at the station. When he got back he told us they would release Benjamin; if we were lucky he would be free early the next morning. The experience was well documented by Benjamin in an English comp assignment called "Last Week I Was a Criminal."[13]

Mike and I spent the entire night in the hallway of the police department waiting for Benjamin to be released. Finally, hours later, he came through the door. What a relief! I had never experienced anything like this, and I hoped I never would again. We were told to come back, together with Benjamin, the next day.

After this horrible ordeal, Benjamin asked me to come to his apartment, by myself, without Zoë. He wanted to talk to me. Obviously, this was the discussion he had wanted to have the night he was thrown in jail. We sat on the couch, and carefully he tried to explain to me that he thought there was something wrong. He tired very quickly and needed much more sleep than he was used to. He said he had found a bump on his testicle and was afraid it might be cancer. At the time it did not alarm me. I had never heard of testicular cancer and did not even know that type of cancer existed. I comforted him and said that it was probably a cyst, nothing to worry about, and that he needed to see a urologist to have a look at it. I assured him again it would not be anything serious. I explained to him that I myself had had a Bartholin cyst just after he was born and that a minor operation had removed it. We enjoyed the rest of the evening, and before midnight I went back home to be with Mike and Zoë.

Our week in Austin was almost over; it was almost time to fly back to Holland. But before I left, I made sure all the details of Benjamin's ordeal with the police had been taken care of. I went to the West Lake police station where they had booked him to make sure all his outstanding tickets were paid. When I got to the station, they had crossed off the speeding. So Benjamin was right; he never speeded that night. I paid $10 for his car inspection and an outrageous fee of $566.25 because he smoked a cigarette in the cell. In the meantime we heard from the lawyer that Benjamin needed to go to court on May 27. His lawyer also informed us that by that date they probably would not have done anything about the case and that he would likely have to return

---

13.   This story can be found in the addendum at the end of the book.

several times before it was finally dealt with. He said it would probably take up to six months. I promised Benjamin I would be back in Austin on May 26 so that I could be there for him when he needed to be in court. On April 30, Zoë and I returned to Holland.

On Friday evening, May 14, 1999, I had just returned to my apartment in the center of Rotterdam from my consultancy job. Another hectic day with all sorts of system problems was over. Ever since the company had gone "live" on their Enterprise Resource Planning (ERP) system, I had worked long hours.[14] The American team responsible for the implementation had left, and I was the "lucky'" one remaining to take care of support now that the company was up and running on the system. Here I was, back in Holland, again separated from my husband and my son. Why did I ever choose the crazy profession of ERP consultant? I knew it involved lots of traveling, going from place to place, not just in the United States but internationally as well. I did not even like flying!

I threw my shoes off and made myself comfortable, ready to enjoy the weekend. Then the phone rang. It was Benjamin. He told he had gone to see a urologist the day before, in the center of Austin, near where he lived. Blood tests had been done and an ultrasound was made. And now he had received the results. "Mom," he said, "I have cancer. I am diagnosed with testicular cancer."

Silence. It was as if my heart stopped beating; I gasped for air. I was flabbergasted and could not believe my ears. Benjamin must have sensed my concern and tried to comfort me by telling me that the survival rate for testicular cancer was high, approximately 95 percent. The urologist had told him that it was no big deal, that he should have his testicle removed right away, followed by a couple of rounds of chemotherapy, and he would be as good as new before he knew it. He would be able to continue college again after summer. I told Benjamin on the phone that I would return to Austin on the first available flight to be there for him and that I needed to hang up so that I could make flight arrangements.

---

14.   ERP is a term usually used in conjunction with ERP Software, e.g., SAP software, or an ERP system, which is intended to manage all the information and functions of a business or company from shared data stores.

I was devastated, confused. My beautiful son had a deadly disease. How was this possible? I needed to get back to Austin; I needed to be there for my son. I called KLM, the Dutch Royal Airlines, to see if I could fly out the next morning. I was lucky; they did have a seat available. I booked right away on the phone; I would pick up the tickets in the departure hall. Soon after I had hung up, my Dutch friend called, a friend I had known since elementary school and with whom I had shared a lot of the good and bad times. This friend would drop me during the most difficult time of my life. As soon as I picked up the phone, I started crying. She said, "What's wrong? What's wrong?" I could not say a word. She kept screaming, demanding to know what was wrong. Finally the words came out. "Benjamin just called, and they diagnosed … he has cancer!"

"Oh my God, this can't be true … this can't be true …" My friend herself had lost her brother to cancer only a year before. She understood how I felt. I remembered her talking about her brother, how this awful disease had taken his life, how he had wasted away toward the end. How awfully thin he had become, how he had suffered. Was this what was awaiting Benjamin? I could not believe it. He was only twenty-one years old! None of this could be true. While on the phone with her, I told her something I had never ever told anyone in my life.

When Benjamin was just a baby I always felt there was something wrong, that he was not well. I had nightmares that when I picked him up underneath his little arms, he would slip right through my hands, as if I could not hold on to him. I experienced those feelings over and over. However, as he grew to be a normal, healthy baby, the feelings disappeared, and I never thought about them again—until now, until this telephone conversation. My friend listened to what I had to say, and she replied, "Those feelings, the nightmares, had nothing to do with time. This could be anywhere in life."

We talked a little longer, but I felt an urgency to hang up; I was restless and needed to get going as soon as possible to pack all my stuff. Because I was in an apartment that belonged to my employer, I had to get all my personal belongings out of there, as I did not know if I would be back at all. I called Zoë and told her that Benjamin had been diagnosed with cancer. It was a shock all over again, and she was devastated. Of course she understood that I had to return to Austin immediately and that I had to be with Benjamin. She promised to help me get the stuff out of the apartment and see me off the next morning.

Although I needed to be rested for the ten-hour flight, I could not sleep. Instead I sat behind my computer and surfed the Internet to learn about testicular cancer. How come I was not aware of this disease? How come young men were not made aware of this cancer, like women were made aware of breast cancer? I found a couple of pages, but not too many. I read as much as I could to find out what the risks were, what treatments were available.

I can't remember my flight back to Austin, can't remember what my thoughts were, how I was dealing with it all. I only know that Benjamin was waiting for me at the airport. He stood there while I came through the gate. He looked good, very handsome, not like a young man who had a deadly disease. It all seemed so unreal. He drove me to my house in South Austin and dropped me off. I agreed I would come to his apartment the next day, and we would discuss what action needed to be taken. I walked into the house; Mike was surprised to see me. I had not called him to let him know that I was coming. He was wondering why I was back, and I told him that Benjamin had been diagnosed with cancer. He was devastated.

The next day I drove up to Benjamin's apartment. Benjamin suggested we walk to the park and have our discussion there. The park was very close, just across the road. In the park he asked me, regardless of how odd this might all sound to me, to respect his choices and to support him in his decisions. He then made it clear to me that he was not going to follow the conventional therapies for his cancer. He said he wanted to follow alternative therapies. I was shocked. I did not know anything about alternative therapies, nor did I know much about conventional therapies, for that matter. It was obvious that Benjamin had already looked into several options. He had also bought a couple of books on the matter. I warned him that if he chose to take the path of alternative medicine that if he changed his mind later, it might be too late to reverse the disease with conventional medicine. I tried not to sound too worried, but I was extremely worried. I wanted to be there for him; I wanted to support him as much as I could, but I had never thought for one minute that he would not follow the advice his urologist had given him. We spoke some more about the disease and how devastating it can be. I told him that dying of cancer could be a terrible death. He was taking a big risk by turning away from conventional treatment. But Benjamin said that was the choice he had made. He said further, "If in two years I have survived this disease, it will be reason to celebrate; however, if I die within the next two years, it will still be reason to celebrate. It will mean that whatever my task on this earth might have been, I will have fulfilled that task."

What could I do? He was an adult, over twenty-one, and I could not make him do anything. He was responsible for his own decisions, for his own actions. He had to accept the repercussions. I promised him I would be there for him, that I would support him, no matter what. But my heart was aching. Benjamin, meanwhile, felt he had been given a chance to heal himself. He wrote in his journal: "So far, it has been one big positive experience. Healing is not determined by the amount of years you live, but to be at peace when your time does come."

The following days, Benjamin and I looked at all the alternatives out there. We visited bookstores all over town to check out the books on alternative treatments for cancer. I could not believe my eyes—I would have never known that there were so many unorthodox therapies if Benjamin hadn't brought them to my attention. We bought several books, including *An Alternative Medicine Definitive Guide to Cancer*[15], which I thought was the best. It was a book with more than a thousand pages on how cancer can be reversed using clinically proven complementary and alternative therapies. A total of thirty-seven top physicians explained their treatments in this book.

The first couple of days that third week in May 1999, we read everything there was to be read. First we checked out all the pages on the "Cancer Industry." Could what was printed there in black and white be true? Had the conventional cancer establishment deceived us? Had we, the public, been kept in the dark? Reading through the pages, it was obvious that money had a lot to do with it. Cancer is medicine's biggest business. In the United States alone, over $1 trillion has been spent on treatment, research, and indirect costs since President Nixon declared the War on Cancer almost forty years before. Yet very little had been accomplished. The number of people still dying of cancer each year is

---

15.   W. John Diamond, MD, and W. Lee Cowden, MD, *Alternative Medicine Definitive Guide to Cancer*. Tiburon, CA: Future Medicine Publishing, 1997.

staggering. It was obvious that the Cancer Industry had not been very successful.

The first part of the book described successful cancer treatments from twenty-three alternative physicians. I went through those chapters one by one. Then I came across one chapter that described a clinic in New York state that had been very successful in reversing testicular cancer, without deadly chemical drugs like chemotherapy, using instead alternative, natural methods—methods not damaging to the body. I became very exited as I read the pages over and over. I realized if Benjamin wanted to go the alternative route—and I had promised him I would support him, regardless of whether I agreed with him or not—this clinic was probably his best bet. This was it. We needed to contact the doctor running this center.

On May 18, 1999, we called the Center for Complementary Medicine in Suffern, New York, after we had carefully looked at all the alternatives. We spoke to Dr. Reynolds of the Center, who requested we fax Benjamin's medical records, particularly the results from the urologist, so the Center staff could evaluate the details. The results from the urologist showed that his AFP[16] tumor marker, a substance that is found in blood, was 270; the beta-HCG[17] marker was 690. An elevated level of a tumor marker can indicate cancer. In the meantime Benjamin was advised to live as healthily as possible, meaning that he should eat whole foods and lots of vegetables, preferably juiced, and drink four to six ounces of vegetable juices, including two to three carrots. He was advised to stop smoking immediately, both cigarettes and any other substances. They would call us back once they had looked at his medical records.

Toward the end of that week, the Center called us back and informed us that they were willing to accept Benjamin as their patient. However, before he could begin treatment, Benjamin needed to have his testicle removed. Because we were living in Texas, he advised us to go to the MD Anderson Hospital in Houston.

However, this was something Benjamin absolutely refused to do. He said so to the Center, and they regretfully informed us that in that case

16.   AFP stands for alpha-fetoprotein. Normal AFP levels are <5–10 ng/ml (nanograms per milliliter).
17.   HCG stands for human chorionic gonadotropin. A normal level for beta-HCG is < 5. Anything higher than 25 ng/ml is considered elevated.

they were unable to help us any further. We were back at square one. It felt as if we had wasted a whole week. We had to start searching for a capable clinic all over again. I began to get very nervous about all this. Every minute counted; we could not afford to lose time. Wasn't everyone always told how important time is when you are a cancer patient—the sooner treatment is started, the better the survival chances?

As we began researching alternative doctors and clinics again, I tried to persuade Benjamin to have his testicle removed. Both Mike and I begged him to have the operation done and the tumor removed. It had not only been suggested by the Center in Suffern, but also by his urologist. But no matter how hard I tried to convince him, Benjamin would not listen. "Nobody is cutting parts out of my body," he would say. Benjamin respected human life tremendously and felt that removing important organs was not the way to go. He believed the body could heal itself and that there was no need to do damage to your body. Not until after Benjamin had died and I found his writings did I begin to understand why he had behaved the way he did.

During the early days after Benjamin learned he had cancer, he wrote that he was blessed. He wrote that he had struggled with fear for eternity and that the only way to bliss is through fear; before you experience security you must experience insecurity, and before you can heal you must hurt. In certain cultures it is believed one must overcome serious illness to be able to become a shaman or medicine man. Benjamin's believe was similar. In order to heal others, you must first have healed yourself. He wrote that to him, his task was clear. Once he had overcome his illness, his task would be to help others to do the same. Benjamin wrote in his journal that his view on life had changed these past few days. His will to live had become stronger. Becoming knowledgeable about alternative cancer treatments and sharing that information with several people made him feel good. He felt he was making a difference and felt happy. Again he wrote that his cancer was a blessing.

Then unexpectedly, the following Sunday, on May 23, we received a phone call from Dr. Schachter from the Center for Complementary Medicine. Dr. Schachter, MD, the Center's director, is a magna cum laude graduate of Columbia College of Physicians and Surgeons. He said he had been thinking about Benjamin the past couple of days and was willing, after all, to treat him, if we were prepared to sign a release saying that we would not sue him, should the treatment be unsuccessful. Apparently, he was not allowed to offer any alternative treatment if Benjamin had not first gone the conventional route. We were only too eager to accept his offer. Suing is not part of the Dutch culture, and we really had no problem with signing such a document. A heavy load fell off my shoulders, and I was relieved that Benjamin was going to be accepted for treatment by the clinic of his choice.

We made arrangements to fly to New York and receive treatment. We flew on Tuesday, June 1, from Austin to Newark. We arrived in Newark around eleven thirty in the morning, and a limo picked us up to take us to the Holiday Inn in Suffern. The hotel was a two-minute walk from the Center. I was very worried about Benjamin and how far the cancer had already spread. He had told me that he had not slept the past couple of nights and that he was experiencing backaches. During the flight he was very uncomfortable, and it hurt me tremendously to see him in pain. Nothing is worse for a mother than seeing her child suffer. You want to make it better, take the pain away, but you can't.

On the day we arrived in Suffern, we were scheduled for two hours of medical examination at the clinic between 3:00 and 5:00 PM. Anita, the receptionist, had asked us to be there at 2:00 PM for administrative purposes. Dr. Schachter was placing Benjamin in a very intensive two-week program, especially since Benjamin had chosen not to have surgery. The main treatment involved Amygdalin, which Benjamin received intravenously. Over the years, there have been many conflicting theories about the efficacy of Amygdalin, but regardless of what had been written about it by opponents of alternative medicine, Benjamin felt comfortable with his choice of Amygdalin.

Benjamin visited the clinic every day for a couple of hours while he got his various IVs. Now and then he got a bit frustrated with all those needles that were poked into him. His moods seemed to swing. During his time in Suffern, he recorded in his journal: "At times the feeling of excitement for life leaves me, and death, while I am still young, seems preferable." Every so often he wondered whether he had anything to say in the choice between life and death. Was it his choice? Was it his will that decided whether to live or not? "And if I do not survive the cancer, does this mean my desire to die is bigger?" he asked himself. "Or is it up to a higher power, a bigger universe that decides whether my time is up? I know that when I die I have fulfilled my task on this earth. I know what my task is in this world when I live. The rest is not important."

After his IVs were completed, the remainder of the day was ours, and since we were there in the state of New York, we might as well make the best of it. To be able to go places and do some sightseeing, I decided to rent a car. It was nice to spend some days together with Benjamin, without any other family members there—just the two of us—to do some bonding with my son. He was now twenty-one years old; I really enjoyed Benjamin's company. He was no longer a teenager but a young adult who knew what he wanted in life. He had become a handsome, well-mannered, and respectful young man. I was proud of my son.

The area we were in was beautiful, densely wooded with big, tall, strong trees. The weather was nice, and it was a pleasure to visit several places. We had dinner together at different restaurants; we went to the malls, to movie theaters. We looked in tons of little unique stores. These little towns were so different from the ones in Texas; there was so much more to see and admire. Now that Benjamin was receiving treatment from a very capable doctor, I felt less tense, and I had strong hopes that everything would be all right. Benjamin was somewhat indifferent. He was content with himself, with life and with death. He wrote: "If my destiny is to die young, then so be it. If my destiny is to overcome this illness and help others to do the same, so be it. … We all have to take the bitter with the sweet; there is no way around that. … I wish for my family and the people around me to come to some of these understandings."

During the weekend we decided to drive down to New Jersey to visit his grandmother. Nana lived with her daughter Paula and Paula's son Brett. Benjamin's granddad had already passed away several years before. Because we had spent most of our lives in the Netherlands, Benjamin had only visited with them a couple of times and did not really know them that well. Last time we had visited them was in 1996, already three years past. I had called them earlier in the week from the hotel and asked them if they were going to be home during the coming weekend and if it was okay that Benjamin and I dropped by. Of course, we were very welcome. Nana always enjoys having her family around, and she made us more than welcome. She insisted we stay with here and would not let us spend the night in a nearby hotel. I can't remember whether I told them on the phone the reason we were in Suffern, or whether we actually told them that Benjamin had cancer during our visit. Regardless, they were devastated by the news.

It was good to see them again. While at Nana's we enjoyed the nice summer weather. We all sat outside and caught up on all that had happened during the past couple of years. We hadn't seen each other for so long. At the same time I could tell that we all were very worried about Benjamin. Paula was very worried about Benjamin's decision to go the alternative route. She really tried to persuade him to believe in the expertise and knowledge of the conventional doctors. She mentioned how a friend of hers had cancer but was now in remission, thanks to chemotherapy. But no matter what anybody said, Benjamin had made up his mind and was only going to use alternative therapies.

After an enjoyable weekend at Nana's we drove back up to Suffern for Benjamin's second week of treatment. Before we knew it the two weeks of medical care were over, and we were almost ready to go back to Texas again. Benjamin could not wait to get home. These past weeks had been good for him. The Amygdalin IVs he had received had stopped the backaches. Dr. Schachter had found a holistic doctor in Austin who was willing to administer the daily Amygdalin IVs Benjamin needed. I was relieved. At least he could continue his therapy. Everybody at the clinic had been so very nice to us. Shirley, a lady at the clinic's front desk, told Benjamin something that touched him. She said he had a sparkle or shine about him, as if he knew something most of us don't. Through the years, and especially the last years before his death, several people had told me what an extraordinary young man my son was—so respectful and well mannered. He left a very positive impression; he stood out. Benjamin made a note to send the people at the clinic a thank-you card when he got back home and to let them know how he was doing.

We had decided to visit New York City before flying back. We stayed in a hotel at the airport. This would be our first visit ever to New York. Neither Benjamin nor myself had ever visited the actual city. Of course we had flown via the New York airport several times in the past years, going back and forth to Europe. We were exited about visiting. Most of his life Benjamin had wanted to come here. The first thing we did was visit the World Trade Center. From there we had an awesome view of Manhattan. It was really amazing. When we were back "down under," we decided to go our separate ways. I could not blame Benjamin—after all, he was a twenty-one-year-old young man. He did not want to spend the entire day with his mother, even though we had bonded and grown in our relationship during our two weeks' stay in Suffern and had enjoyed each other's company. Benjamin went downtown and got to know some interesting people, who invited him back to New York anytime he wanted. I decided to take the ferry to Ellis Island. Through this small island in New York Harbor, millions of emigrants entered the United States over a century ago. I enjoyed visiting the site and reading up on all the history that took place on Ellis Island. Benjamin and I agreed to meet again later that afternoon at the World Trade Center and take a taxi back to the hotel. The next morning we flew back to Austin.

The following week we made arrangements with Dr. Vladimir Rizov, MD, the holistic doctor Dr. Schachter had found for us, and scheduled appointments for his daily IVs. I went along with Benjamin to Dr. Rizov's practice and stayed the entire time while he was receiving the Amygdalin IVs. I felt that was the least I could do. Apart from that, I felt pretty helpless, wishing I could do more, could take his pain away. I had ordered the vials from the same place that Dr. Schachter had ordered them. Then, after a couple of weeks of treatments, out of the blue, Benjamin decided he was not going to go to Dr. Rizov anymore. He was going to try a different approach; he was going to just stick with Essiac tea. [18]

His decision scared me stiff. What made him stop with the treatment all of a sudden? Why was he being so obstinate? Why was he experimenting with different alternative therapies? Did he not understand that cancer was not an innocent cold or something minor but a life threatening disease? I was so worried; it made me feel sick to

---

18.   Essiac was first promoted as a cancer treatment in the 1920s. The four main herbs that make up Essiac tea are burdock root, slippery elm inner bark, sheep sorrel, and Indian rhubarb root. The original formula is believed to have its roots with the native Canadian Ojibwa Indians. Cynthia Olsen, *Essiac: A Native Herbal Cancer Remedy*, 2nd ed. (Twin Lakes, WI: Lotus Press, 1998).

my stomach. But what could I do? He was an adult—nothing I said or begged of him made any difference. Benjamin was Benjamin, and he did what he thought he needed to do. He explained to me that he believed the human body was capable of healing itself. He approached his cancer treatment with the guiding principle of the Hippocratic Oath, which states, "First, do no harm." Since chemotherapy harmed the body, he did not want to do it. He also felt that removing parts of the body showed disrespect toward the human body. All I could do was stand by, watch, and be supportive. During this period a young man Benjamin's age in my birth town had just died from cancer, and Benjamin began wondering how long it was before he would breathe his last breath. "Ready for death? Almost," he wrote. "When I am twenty-two?" he asked himself.

While he was relying on only the Essiac tea for his treatment, he also experienced a very out of the ordinary happening. Benjamin attended a ceremony of the Sioux Indians in Rockdale, Texas. One evening, Benjamin had to spend time in the sweat tent to get rid of his toxins. This needed to be done in preparation for what was coming. After midnight Benjamin and some others sat in the "medicine circle" around the campfire. This is, according to the Sioux Indians, the holy fire. Benjamin was given peyote, a small, spineless cactus, to eat and some peyote tea to drink. Native Americans used the plant for its curative properties. Peyote is extremely bitter, and most people are nauseated. Benjamin had to throw up. This was good and seen as getting rid of all your emotional and physical garbage. The vomit was quickly buried, and after that he had to eat and drink more peyote to fill up the empty space that now existed with the good. This went on the entire night, and Benjamin described this spiritual experience as if a load fell from his shoulders. His backache seemed to have disappeared, and he had a feeling of pure knowledge and insight—everything seemed very clear. In the morning he was served fresh food, and everything tasted excellent. Everything was beautiful and good. The next couple of days Benjamin felt strong and fit, and he looked good. Perhaps this spiritual event happened during the short period that he was very upbeat and optimistic about his disease. He was not going to let it ruin his life. But that did not last very long, because a while later Benjamin's backache returned, and the pain seemed worse than before.

Benjamin was still living by himself in the small apartment just off Mopac, the apartment he had shown me so proudly earlier that year, before he knew he had cancer, when he was so excited about his future. I had asked him several times to come and stay with me so that I could look after him, but he refused. No matter how I pleaded with him, he was not going to move back in with me. So I went by to see him as much and as frequently as I could; I kept the apartment clean, cooked for him, and made sure that he drank his fruit and vegetable juices. But everything was a struggle. Then one night, when Mike and I were already in bed, the phone rang. It was Benjamin, asking me to come over as soon as possible. He sounded desperate, very stressed. I got up, dressed as quickly as I could, and jumped in the car, only to find that I was nearly out of gas. I was just hoping that I could make it to the nearest gas station and that they would be still open in the middle of the night.

When I reached Benjamin's apartment I found him in terrible pain. He could barely sit straight and begged me to make the pain go away. I was devastated, unable to do anything, feeling totally helpless. Painkillers did not work; nothing helped. There was just this awful pain in his lower back. At one point, he suddenly jumped on his bike and raced back and forth in the streets near his apartment, trying to get rid of the pain, or perhaps trying to forget he had a pain. Exhausted, he came back into the apartment where I was waiting for him.

I can't remember how he made it through the night or how I got home, but the next day I managed to get him to my house. I had visited him again, and for some reason we went back to Bernoulli Drive in my car. Perhaps it was to have dinner. I'm not sure what the reason was. At home, Mike and myself discussed the situation with him, and again we talked to him about having the tumor removed in the Anderson Hospital in Houston, as was recommended by Dr. Schachter. But again, Benjamin would not listen. He did not want to even discuss the possibility. In the meantime, his health was deteriorating. He was no longer receiving the daily IVs or taking all the supplements that he was supposed to take. He was in terrible pain most of the time. What was he thinking? What made him choose this path, a path of unproven therapies, a path so different from what was recommended? I could not understand his choices. My son Benjamin was a highly intelligent human being, always had been the best at school. What made him behave like this? I questioned him several times, wondering whether it was fear. Was he afraid of an operation; was he afraid of the hospital, the doctors? He claimed he was not.

After dinner, he asked to be taken back to his apartment. Again I asked him to stay with us so that we could properly take care of him, but again he refused. I told him I was not going to drive him back, thinking he would have no choice but to stay with Mike and me. Instead, he said he would walk, and he packed his stuff and walked outside. But he was in too much pain to be able to walk straight. I could not see him suffer the way he was, so in the end I did drive him back to his apartment. Having to leave him there by himself was very painful for me, but what could I do? The only thing I could do was to accept, be supportive, and be there for him whenever he needed me.

Every day that I visited Benjamin, I tried to convince him to go back to the clinic and to get his daily IVs. I bargained with him, pleaded, and begged, anything that I could think of to make him see that he needed to take action; that he needed to take this disease seriously. And every day I felt totally helpless—hopeless, almost. I did not seem to be able to get through to him. I did not know what I could do to make him change his mind.

A couple of weeks later, after talking on the phone one day to his Aunt Susan in New Jersey, he told me that he wanted to move to New Jersey and that he seriously wanted to start working on his health. We would go to New Jersey for six months to concentrate on his well-being. I was relieved and glad. It sounded as though his aunt had been able to talk some sense into him. Susan would become my closest confident over the next nine months.

I was glad about his choice, because it would mean that we would be very close to Dr. Schachter's clinic, within driving distance anyway. I was hopeful that he would go back to Dr. Schachter's clinic and continue his therapy. And my ex-in-laws were in New Jersey. I felt that being close to his grandma, his aunts, and other relatives would offer us a better support system. In Texas we had no direct relatives; it was just Benjamin and myself. All my relatives were in the Netherlands, including his sister, his father. Of course my husband Mike and his relatives were in Texas, but Mike's relatives did not know Benjamin; they did not have an emotional connection with him. I felt we needed the support only direct family members are able to give.

CHAPTER 3

New Jersey

Dying in my belief is called among other things: Upgrading
Note to the dying—
You can always try again
Even after you are dead

Benjamin Hyman

Once Benjamin decided to move to New Jersey, the next thing to do was arrange everything that needed to be arranged for the move. I had decided to move with him and be there for him while he was residing in New Jersey. And because my employer was in Philadelphia, it was convenient for me as well to be in New Jersey. The sad thing was that I had to leave Mike behind again.

The first thing we needed to arrange was for an apartment or house to live in. This was not as simple as it sounded and definitely more difficult than in Austin. In Austin there were tons of apartments for rent. No shortage there. I even considered buying some New Jersey property, if renting was going to be a problem. I contacted several agencies that could help me find a place. It was a bit awkward, as I could not go and check them out. I needed to totally relay on the agencies.

We finally found a furnished two-bedroom apartment in Maple Shade that was available immediately. As this was only going to be temporary, I was not too concerned. I would be able to find something that we really liked once we were in New Jersey. We decided to take all Benjamin's belongings, including his car, with us, as well as some furniture from our home in Austin. Of course, we needed to take all Benjamin's stuff because we had to cancel his rental contract, and we needed to empty the apartment out.

Because the road trip was far too exhausting, Benjamin was flying from Austin to Newark. He flew on Sunday, August 1, 1999. I had arranged for Susan to pick him up from the airport. The plane arrived in Newark at 6:27 PM. I was going to drive a rented truck, loaded with our stuff, and tow Benjamin's car all the way from Austin to New Jersey. Mike had decided to come with me. We figured out it was going to take approximately three days to drive from our home to our destination in New Jersey. We were leaving on Friday, hoping to be in New Jersey Sunday afternoon. We could not afford to take more time, as Mike needed to be back at work the next Monday. He was scheduled to fly back on Sunday evening.

Getting all Benjamin's stuff out of the apartment took some time, but we had help from our neighbors, and everything went relatively smoothly, considering. Then we were ready to hit the road. I was actually looking forward to the trip. We decided to take the nicer route—that is, the more scenic route, through Tennessee, Kentucky, and West Virginia. I had traveled up north plenty of times, but always by plane. This would be a nice change. Besides I got some time just with Mike.

The trip went well. We took turns driving. We decided not to travel through the night but to book into a hotel. Even though we were well rested from staying in hotels during the nights, when we finally arrived in New Jersey, we were pretty exhausted. We had arranged for Shirley and Ben, the couple that was leasing their apartment to us, to meet at a main spot within the local town. Once we met up, they drove in front of us, directing us to the apartment complex in Maple Shade. The truck was left in a parking lot until I found storage space and we could unload the truck. However, that was for later. No need to worry about it yet. We arrived at the apartment, which turned out to be quite a nice place, well maintained and clean. It was fully furnished and had everything we needed, from pots and pans to towels and bedding.

Mike called a cab, which arrived shortly, and he left for the Philadelphia airport. So there I was, by myself in this apartment in this strange, unknown place. I anxiously awaited Benjamin's arrival. I was extremely worried about him. I knew how much pain he was constantly in and how very tiring most activities were for him. I hoped that the plane ride would not have been too exhausting for him.

After a couple of hours my two ex-sisters-in-law and Benjamin arrived safely. I was glad to see them all. Benjamin had survived the trip without too much hassle, but I could tell he was very tired. Both his aunts looked worried. They had not seen Benjamin since our visit to New Jersey at the beginning of June. Almost two months later, they now noticed that his health had deteriorated and that he wasn't looking too good. We chitchatted a bit and caught up on what everybody had been up to. Then it was time for them to leave.

Benjamin and I went to bed early. The next couple of days we were busy arranging all sorts of things. The truck got unloaded and returned to the rental agency. We had to place all our belonging in storage. Benjamin's cousin Jason helped to unload and store all our stuff. No way could we have managed all that work by ourselves, as Benjamin only could help with the smaller stuff—he was too much in pain, but he tried.

The next thing we did was to make an appointment with Dr. Schachter. We visited him on August 9 and enjoyed the drive up to Suffern. The area was so beautiful. It was good to see everyone at the clinic again. The visit itself did not turn out to be such a success. Benjamin was being more obstinate than ever before. He did not want to listen to Dr. Schachter's advice, which was to do vitamin C and hydrogen peroxide therapy intravenously, have nutritional and pharmacologic support, and take additional vitamins. He flat out refused these suggestions. I tried to talk to the young man, but he would not listen and was simply unresponsive. It was one of these occasions whereby he knew it all, and everybody, including the medical professionals, was totally wrong. He was just going to follow his own beliefs. No matter how we all tried, we could not get through to him. I yelled at him out of frustration and told him I was through with him, that if he was going to continue this way he was surely to die. It did not have any impact whatsoever.

Once more I wondered why he was behaving like this; once more I failed to follow his train of thought. The only positive thing that came out of this visit was that he did allow blood tests, and he accepted Dr. Schachter's recommendation of Dr. Magaziner in Cherry Hill, New Jersey, just ten minutes down the road from our home. The clinic in Suffern was a two-hour drive and having a doctor near where we now lived was a blessing.

Dr. Magaziner was going to administer Benjamin's Amygdalin IVs on a daily basis. Benjamin started his IVs at the clinic in Cherry Hill on August 11. The blood results came back from the sample drawn in Austin in late July, and they were not good. The HCG had gone up dramatically. It stood now at 21,900.

Although our apartment in Maple Shade was very comfortable and nice, I started looking for another place; our stuff from Texas was still in storage, and we began missing our personal belongings. Besides, we were expecting a lot of visitors over the next weeks and months. I had finally been able to convince Benjamin's father to come over. I felt he needed to be here with his son. Benjamin needed his support as well. Zoë and Frido also decided to come over to see us rather than going on a European vacation. It would be nice if we had a bigger place with more bedrooms so that they could stay with us rather than having to book hotel rooms.

After only one month in Maple Shade, I found a beautiful three-bedroom townhouse with a loft in Marlton. Besides the house being nice, the area was magnificent as well. It felt as though we were living in a beautiful park, quiet and peaceful, full of tall trees and large ponds. We had our belongings moved into our new home, and we were ready to welcome our visitors.

During the period we had our loved ones over from Europe, Wayne, I, and Benjamin visited an oncologist, Dr. John Garofalo, MD, in Bryn Mawr, Pennsylvania. We had finally been able to persuade Benjamin that he needed to see an oncologist. Dr. Garofalo was picked because Dr. Magaziner told us he was open-minded with regard to alternative therapies. Of course, when we visited him, he tried to persuade Benjamin to go for chemotherapy. He tried to convince Benjamin that testicular cancer was one of the cancers where chemotherapy was very successful and that the success rate was higher than 95 percent. Nevertheless, when Benjamin could not be convinced, he accepted Benjamin's viewpoint and did not push further. He told Wayne and me that all we could do was to provide Benjamin with information, but it was up to him to take action.

During all those months since my return from Holland, I had not been working. Fortunately there had been no new projects, and my employer had been extremely kind to let me stay home and take care of Benjamin. However, now that we were living in New Jersey, very close to my employer, it was expected that I would go into the office once in a while. I was also asked to go to San Diego for a couple of days to attend and participate in a SAP-related exhibition. The idea was to do some networking and see if I could get companies interested in our SAP Consultancy work. I loved San Diego, and the short trip did me good. I was able to visit a very good friend who was from San Diego, whom I had not seen for quite some years. He took me out and showed the town. I was worried about Benjamin, and I did feel guilty that I had to leave him by himself. But he had promised that he would take care of himself, that he would go and see Dr. Magaziner for his IVs and go to eat at his grandma's or Susan's.

Then, starting in September I was assigned to a project just outside of Chicago, which meant I would be traveling again every week, getting on an airplane on Mondays, flying back to Philadelphia on Fridays. The project was to last a few months. I had no choice; I needed to earn a living and could not afford to quit my job. Because I had to go back to work and leave Benjamin by himself during the week, I made an agreement with Susan that she would look after Benjamin when I was not there. She promised she would keep in touch with him every day and make sure he went to his doctor for his daily IVs. She would get him to come over or she would go and see him, whatever he wanted. Susan and I kept in contact mostly via e-mail.

Every night and whenever I got a chance, I would explore the Internet, finding information on cancer and cancer treatments. I came to realize that there were many different ways of treating cancer and that these different treatments had saved lives. So many success stories were out there from cancer survivors. Any kind of therapy or alternative options I could find I would print and save in a binder. I tried to share them with Benjamin. Some options sounded so very promising. It was frustrating not only for me, but for all of us that were close to Benjamin that he was not more proactive. There were so many alternative possibilities out there. It was especially frustrating because he did not want to go the conventional way and insisted on alternative, nonaggressive therapies.

I had supported him when he first told me he was going to treat this disease with alternative methods. So why didn't he grab every possible option that was out there? I just did not understand him. No matter what I said to him, no matter how often I begged him—so many times—it all seemed to have a negative impact on him. What was wrong with him? Perhaps the oncologist was right. All we could do was supply him with information. It was up to him to run with it.

The more we begged him to do something, the more he resisted. Susan had also tried to share and talk to him about his treatment and other choices, but he just shut her down. He did not want to hear, and he would not listen. Susan found him to be very stubborn and single-minded at times. As intelligent as he was, he did not know it all, and he was not willing to listen and learn. She let him know how she felt, that she was frustrated that he wasn't doing enough to get rid of the cancer.

Even though Benjamin had a life-threatening disease, he had still lots of hopes and dreams. He talked about his education. He showed an interest in the Philadelphia College of Art, now that we were living in New Jersey. He talked about enrolling at Temple University in October for the January semester. He wanted to move to the center of the city. He had even gone down to Philadelphia to see some apartments and lofts that were for rent. However, I was deeply concerned about Benjamin because one day he was up, the next day he was down. Sometimes he missed his IV appointments, and it seemed he was not taking the responsibility he should take. How could I let him go to live in Philadelphia under these circumstances? No matter how much I wished the best for him, how much I wished he would be well again, no matter how much research I did, handing him all the information on what options there were out there, it was up to him to take action. I could not force him to do anything.

All that made me so discouraged that at times I felt I could not carry on. I felt like throwing him out of bed on days he stayed in bed all day, when I felt he was wasting his life away, not taking action. But it was his choice. If he wanted to die of this disease, so be it. I told myself I was not going to waste my energy and my own well-being any longer on a battle I could not win. At the time I did not realize he was "protecting" me by not communicating to me that he did not feel well and that when he was in so much pain, he stayed in bed. At times I did not know how he was feeling. What was going on inside of his head? Knowing what he was going through would have helped me tremendously to understand. This not knowing was hard for me. It made me frustrated.

Thank God for Susan. Benjamin did talk with Susan and sometimes confided in her. Susan would then keep me informed. At times he was in good spirits and was open; other times it seemed you could not get through to him. Susan also made sure to remind him when I was traveling and not there that he had to go for his daily IVs. She got him to get a prescription for an MRI. She convinced him it was necessary that he knew what was going on in his body, that he needed to know what was going on with his lymph nodes, especially one in his neck that had started to grow and was becoming visible. Benjamin finally talked about a biopsy. He wanted to have the nodes checked out above his waist and, if necessary, to have some surgically removed. He wanted a complete body scan. He was in so much pain all the time. She reminded him that his main focus was to get well and kick the cancer in the butt. Benjamin agreed to that and said that he had every intention of doing that, but in is own way, at his own pace.

I was glad that Benjamin was beginning to realize he needed proper monitoring and that he could not just guess what was going on in his body. Regretfully, Benjamin did not communicate with me the pains and discomforts he had. I needed to ask him about it, and then when I did, I still did not really know. Didn't he want me to know the truth? Was he worried that I might worry too much?

The end of September approached. We had been in New Jersey for two months. What had we accomplished? Had Benjamin really been concentrating on getting well? I felt we had wasted time; we could have done much more. But I was glad that he was beginning to realize that he needed proper monitoring, that just having his daily IVs was not enough. Soon he was scheduled to have another blood test. Since the last test, Benjamin's tumor markers had decreased, and I was curious to find out if the tumor markers had gone down again this time. Something did not seem to make sense though. If the markers were going down, why were Benjamin's lymph nodes swelling up? Did this mean they were fighting the disease, or was the cancer spreading? If the latter, why were the tumor markers down? If the cancer was spreading, he should have been losing weight, but he was gaining.

Whenever I talked to Benjamin trying to discover why he would not go the conventional way, I always asked whether he was afraid—afraid of the hospital, afraid of an operation. But he always claimed he was not frightened at all. He would remind me of the "do no harm" aspect of the Hippocratic Oath. He also seemed to understand the seriousness of this disease and that it could kill him. Benjamin seemed very fearless and seemed to understand the reality of it all. He said again that if he died from this disease, it would be reason to celebrate, because it meant that his tasks here on earth had been completed. How could he be so calm about this entire ordeal?

Susan felt Benjamin's bravery was false bravery. She felt that he wanted to seem accepting of his disease and of any fate that might come with it. But at times the vulnerable, fearful young man was evident. For me, this whole ordeal was a nightmare and an emotional roller coaster. This is what Benjamin wrote at the time:

> For a while I was quite sure I was getting better. Soon to be cancer-free! Now I am not so sure anymore. The large lymph nodes in my neck and the occasional pain in the left side of my head make me fear it has reached my brain. I am going to have a MRI or CAT scan done to find out what is happening inside me. The HCG tumor makers were looking so promising though. They went from 22,000 to 16,000 to 13,000 to 6,400 over a period of nine weeks. I guess the only thing I can do is to continue with my treatments and anticipate the outcome. Which is one of the two: live or die. Ultimately this is beyond anything I can do, as I believe

when your time has truly come, it is out of your hands. I am
at peace with whatever destiny has planned for me.

Although Benjamin had written that he wanted a biopsy and that he
wanted an MRI or CAT scan, later that year, in December, he changed
his mind.

Beginning in October, I had to return to Vernon Hills, near
Chicago. This time I had to stay a couple of weeks, because we were
in the middle of implementing the system. I would even have to work
during the weekends. I was not pleased with it and dreaded being away
for so long, leaving Benjamin. On the other hand, it was not too bad,
because his best friend Klaas from Holland expected to visit us soon.
So while I was away in Vernon Hills, he would have Klaas around. Also
I could count on Susan. She was always willing to drop by and make
sure he was okay.

Mike was coming to visit the first weekend of October, before I
had to fly out on Monday morning. We had not seen each other for
over two months now. I picked him up early on Saturday morning. We
enjoyed each other's company. We visited Atlantic City and did some
sightseeing around Marlton. It was a nice break, and it helped me not to
worry about Benjamin for a couple of days. Benjamin, in the meantime,
was supposed to get his blood results, but he had forgotten. He told me
he felt that the lymph nodes in his neck had gone down some, and he
confirmed that he was going to have a lymph node biopsy. He seemed
in good spirit. Maybe this was because Klaas would be there soon.

The couple of days with Mike flew by, and before I knew it, it was
Monday; I was back at work in Vernon Hills. Benjamin called me that
Monday evening to let me know he had gone to pick up the blood test
results. His tumor markers had gone down to 858. That was wonderful
news. Earlier that day he had stopped by Susan's after his IV. They were
both ecstatic. Benjamin was one happy young man. The Laetrile IVs
were working! What we had read on the Web was all true. The Laetrile
was like a natural chemotherapy, without all the dangerous side effects.
Since July the tumor markers had dropped from over 21,000 all the way
down to 858. It was amazing that they had dropped so much, especially
because Benjamin had recently gone only three times a week to get his

IVs rather than five times. The other odd thing was that he was still not feeling good. He was still in pain all the time.

I was beginning to become very skeptical of doctors and oncologists. Here we had living proof that the tumor markers had gone down dramatically, yet his oncologist kept on pushing for Benjamin to go for chemotherapy, even though Benjamin was gaining weight. He did not want to believe that the Laetrile was working, and rather than working with us, trying to find out where the pain came from, he kept saying he has never seen alternative methods work and he never would. If only oncologists and doctors would be more open and not be so close-minded, we could perhaps one day find a true cure for cancer, without having to use all the deadly toxins that are used today by the conventional medical professionals.

The fact that the tumor markers were down so much gave Benjamin hope; he was even considering having the tumor removed in the near future. Susan had also strongly suggested that he have the tumor in his testicle removed. She said she believed he would, and he finally seemed to have agreed with her, but for now he was anxiously awaiting the arrival of his friend Klaas.

Away from home in a hotel in Vernon Hills, I began to realize that I was getting tired of living out of a suitcase, and I really wanted to stay put and not fly all over the place. I was ready to move home to Texas. These past months had drained a lot of energy out of me; they had been an emotional, wild ride with unpredictable destinations. I cannot begin to describe how I felt during that period—the denial, the agony. Seeing your child, your baby, suffering, not knowing whether he will beat this disease, whether he will live, makes your heart sink into your shoes. Most of the time I thought he would be all right, that he would defeat the disease. But deep down, did I really know for sure? While in the hotel in Vernon Hills I did more research on the Web and stayed up until early hours, reading up on all sorts of stories from guys who had testicular cancer. Lance Armstrong, apparently, walked around with an enlarged testicle for three years before he finally went to see a doctor. By then it had already spread to his lungs and brain. Thank God Benjamin's lungs were clear.

Perhaps because the last blood results were so positive, or perhaps because Susan had been successful convincing him, Benjamin decided to have a biopsy done on his neck tumor. Because I was in Vernon Hills, Susan drove him to the hospital in Bryn Mawr, where Dr. Maged S. Khoory, MD, performed the biopsy. Benjamin had been very nervous about the biopsy and did not know what to expect. Perhaps he was worried that the outcome would be negative, that the cancer had spread to his lymph nodes. But the biopsy report we received back said that it showed a collection of what appeared to be benign cells, and, more significantly, tissue fluid was obtained with it. It did not look like embryonal cell carcinoma. In other words, it did not look like cancer. That was extremely good news. The tumor seemed to be benign. Benjamin was so relieved, as we all were. Shortly after his biopsy he also had an ultrasound of his abdomen and his neck done locally, in Cherry Hill.

In mid-October, Klaas arrived from the Netherlands. It was his first trip to the United States. I was sorry I was not there to pick him up with Benjamin because of my work in Vernon Hills, but I would be home the following weekend and have the opportunity to be with them both. Before Klaas arrived, I had asked Benjamin whether he had ever informed Klaas that he was diagnosed with cancer earlier that year. He had not, because he wanted to tell him in person. Apparently Klaas was in shock when he was told, and he did not really know how to react to it all. His best friend had a deadly disease!

Benjamin seemed happy during the period Klaas was visiting. They went out together, dropped by Susan's, went bowling. They visited New York together during the weekend I was back from my work in Vernon Hills. I dropped them off in Trenton at the train station, and they took the train from there to New York. Before they left Benjamin had received his ultrasound back, I combed it thoroughly during the weekend and looked up every term in the medical dictionary online to make sure I understood the description fully. The report did not say anything, really. It talked about a soft tissue mass in his abdomen. The tumor in his neck showed up as a soft tissue abnormality. I had good faith that there was nothing there, apart from the noncancerous fluid that was found during the biopsy. During the weekend Benjamin's oncologist, Dr. Garofalo, called me. He felt that Benjamin was thinking too lightly about this all and that he should really go the conventional way. He told me that he had never ever seen alternative medicine work and that Benjamin had been misinformed. That he should really come to see him more often and not go to Dr. Magaziner. He said that Benjamin could die from this disease. I told him that Benjamin and I were very much aware of the fact that he could die from it and we were very much informed, both about the conventional and alternative therapies. We, and in particular I, had spend night after night looking up anything and everything we could find about testicular cancer and cancer in general. I also said that I would pass his suggestions along to Benjamin, but I reminded him that I could not force Benjamin to come more often.

Klaas and Benjamin returned from New York. They had a wonderful time. They had stayed in a first-class hotel and, especially for Klaas, that had been an experience. During their stay in New York they had also visited a health fair. Benjamin was very much into everything to do with health, good food, and nature itself. During their visit they bumped into an older Native American. This wise man told Benjamin that he had a very old soul. Later, after Benjamin passed, I would discover the significance of that statement.

When they returned to our rented townhouse in Marlton, I was fortunate to spend a couple of days with Benjamin and Klaas before I had to go back to Vernon Hills. It was good to see Klaas again; it amazed me how good he looked. Inside, I was jealous of how well he looked. Benjamin should look well and healthy. He was the same age as Klaas and deserved a healthy life, a life without the worries and burden he was now carrying. My heart ached for him. During the conversations we had, Benjamin expressed his desire to return to Austin. He wanted to go back to continue with his studies. Apparently studying in Philadelphia was no longer an option for him. Although I am not certain as to what changed his mind, I believe he was missing his friends and the social life he had in Austin.

While I was in Vernon Hills, Susan e-mailed me almost daily, keeping me informed of what was going on with Benjamin. "He is over-tired, needs a good night sleep," she wrote. He was probably overdoing it and going out of his way to accommodate Klaas. My work as a consultant was beginning to get to me. I had been working extremely long hours, sometimes until six in the morning. I decided that I did not want to travel any longer. I began to long to return to Austin, just like Benjamin. In Austin Mike and I had a home. Benjamin could stay with us, and if I was not going to travel anymore, I would be able to take care of him on a daily basis.

When I returned from Vernon Hill, Klaas had gone home, and Benjamin complained that he was not feeling well because of the constant pain. Apparently the painkillers he had been taking for the past couple of months were no longer working very well. It sounded as though he needed something stronger. What was causing the constant pain? Why was he feeling so awful most of the time, while his tumor markers were down and he was gaining weight? Was it because of the drugs? Were side effects acting up?

Again I tried to convince him to have the tumors removed, especially since it seemed the pains were getting worse. No matter how hard I tried, he did not seem to make plans to do so. He would do it at his own pace, if he ever did. It was hard to understand what he was thinking. One minute he would be willing to listen and agreed with the suggestions made; the next he would just let you ramble on and shut you out. Didn't he understand that it was not just he that was suffering, but also his close friends, his relatives? All we wanted was for Benjamin to become healthy again, to be happy and live a very long life. I hoped he would go for another blood test soon. In the meantime I was checking out the testicular cancer Web site to find out which were the best hospitals for surgery to remove the tumors in his body. I was hoping that once we were back in Texas, he would indeed have the tumors removed. I prayed he would make the right decisions and move forward. He could be such a healthy person, with so much potential, if he only would do everything in his power to make that happen.

But not matter how much I wanted him to have the tumors removed I realized that only he had the power. He was in charge of it all. All I or anyone else could do was to remind and inform him. Conversations with Benjamin could be very tiresome and frustrating, especially when he did not do enough to my thinking to get well. At times he would not go for his IVs and only take one B-17 pill—hardly enough to battle cancer with. He knew how serious this disease was, so why was he acting like this? Was he being obstinate to annoy me? I did not understand his train of thought at all. Why could I not get through to him? Thank God for Susan. She seemed to be able to have better conversations with him than I could. Was it because I was his mother and he wanted to protect his mother, or so he thought? Susan told him she would feel a lot better if he made a plan of action to get better. So he promised her that he would start to take three B-17 pills and would increase the pills by one a day until he could take twelve B-17 pills in one day. This dose would exceed the amount of medicine he was receiving in the IVs. He would also incorporate all the other medicines, along with the Essiac tea. When he was back in Austin he would find a surgeon that he could trust and have the tumor removed from his neck.

Neither Susan nor I could understand his passive, low-key handling of the disease. So far his approach had not made him better. He would not listen to anyone, only to his own irrational, idealistic rules, which it seemed at the time he made up as he went along. I tried not to get too upset about his approach for now. As long as he realized that he needed to take larger quantities of the B-17 every day, I was willing to give his new strategy a chance. We just had to wait until his next blood test to see whether his new approach for attacking this disease would work. It really was the only thing I could do: give him a chance, even if what he was doing would not expedite ridding his body of the cancer.

I knew that Susan disagreed with that approach; she was fearful that he would get worse unless he became more proactive. She felt that I should be much tougher with him. I should insist or make him to do it our way. But Benjamin was an adult, and there was no way I could make him do anything. In the past I had begged, screamed, yelled at him, all at no avail. I could jump up and down and then throw myself to the floor, but nothing could change Benjamin's way of thinking, change his way of doing this. When I look back now, sometimes I wish I had done more. However, when I look at the situation logically, I realize that I couldn't have done anything more than I did, and I see that my wishes simply reflect my love for Benjamin. When we visited Dr. Schachter, Benjamin bluntly refused to do what he had requested of him. There was just no way I could have forced my grown son to follow the advice given him.

Susan was right, though. We had come to New Jersey to get well and receive good medical attention, yet now we were talking about getting back to Austin. It was ridiculous. She was extremely unhappy with how things had transpired to date. She realized that I had to deal with everything all day, every day, and that it must be hard on me. At the same time she felt that if I had asserted myself, Benjamin would have listened and done all I wanted him to do. She was wrong there. No matter whether I was assertive or not, Benjamin would have done it his way. We all just felt so helpless. We did not know what to say or what to do anymore. I had tried every method to get through to him and could not offer any more options. There had been so much turmoil and chaos where Benjamin was concerned—perhaps being in familiar surroundings with Mike would help me cope better. The only thing to do was to return home and try to pick up my life, to move forward and to start taking care of myself. It was now up to Benjamin to decide whether he wanted to get well or whether he wanted to die from this disease. I was burned out; the torment inside me became unbearable.

CHAPTER 4

Back to Texas

How come sometimes it is so hard to believe in the positive, when believing the negative is so easy?

Benjamin Hyman

Klaas had gone back home. Benjamin and I were ready to move back to Texas and would do so before Thanksgiving. We were returning to Austin before the original six months were over. Three months earlier, Benjamin had decided he wanted to move north to New Jersey, as he wanted to seriously work on his health and beat this awful disease. He had wanted to be close to his relatives and to Dr. Schachter. But what had become of that goal? Had he accomplished his objective? Hardly, I felt, but Benjamin probably saw it differently. Yes, he was a bit better than when we had first come to New Jersey three months before, but by no means had he kicked the cancer in the butt. He still had a very rough road ahead.

There I was again, making arrangements to move. I was becoming a *zigeuner*, a gypsy, traveling back and forth, not staying put in one place for very long. This time I was not going to bother packing up everything myself. I contacted a removal company, and they were going to pack and transport everything back to Austin, including Benjamin's car. Mike came to help me with the details; he and I would drive my Jeep back to Austin. This time we would not have to haul a trailer with Benjamin's car behind it. I anticipated the trip to be more enjoyable than the one that brought us here. Benjamin would fly back, and he had already made arrangements for his friends to pick him up. Perhaps this had been one of the reasons why he decided he wanted to go back to Austin: He was missing his friends, his social life. While we had been in New Jersey, he had not made any friends. No wonder really, because all that kept him busy was this awful disease, visiting his doctor on almost a daily basis. He carried a burden a young man his age should not have to carry.

Benjamin flew back on Monday, November 22, and arrived safely. The same night he went out to dinner with friends. Mike and I left Marlton that Monday around 1:00 PM. The movers had things packed before we knew it, and then we were on the road back home.

A three-day drive lay ahead of us. This time our trip was somewhat more relaxed than when we drove up to New Jersey. It was autumn, and the countryside was beautiful with trees in full autumn colors. Too bad we could not afford to stay in many places along the way. I made a promise to myself that one day when time was not an issue I would revisit the area. We arrived in Austin Thursday morning—Thanksgiving.

Benjamin had been going for his IVs again once he was back in Austin. He had also had another blood test, but the results were not positive. The tumor markers had gone up again. They were back to 2,100. Not good ... but at least we knew that the IVs had controlled the cancer in the past. While it was possible that the cancer had begun to develop a resistance to the Laetrile, he needed to keep up with the IVs to continue to try and force the tumor markers down to a normal level. The pills alone were not (yet) enough. Benjamin was in good spirits, and he was doing what he needed to do: getting his IVs and taking the pills. I was going to contact the M. D. Anderson Cancer Center in Houston for information. I sincerely hoped I would be able to convince Benjamin now to have the tumors taken out. I also intended to contact Dr. Joseph

Gold[19] or his Institute about the hydrazine sulfate[20] I had ordered while in New Jersey. I wanted to see if he could take these pills together with the narcotics, as Benjamin really wanted to get off painkillers.

In December 1999, I was trying to organize things in Austin. Benjamin's car and the moving truck had arrived a few days ago. I had not realized we had collected that much stuff in New Jersey. Our garage was totally packed. Sorting out all that stuff would keep me busy for some time. Benjamin was staying with us at Bernoulli Drive. He was already back into his routines; he had scheduled a Tai Chi lesson and gone for IVs. I had not had a chance to communicate with him much, so I did not really know how he was feeling. He told me, however, he was doing the IVs and taking additional supplements, such as vitamin C, enzymes, and shark oil. He didn't mention having the tumors removed or seeing an oncologist here in Austin. I was going to have to hang in there a while and try not to worry too much. If Benjamin was not going to come around, I was going to confront him. For now he seemed in good spirits. I just wished he would put on some weight. He seemed awfully thin.

During this period Benjamin wrote: "Life is truly beautiful, death must be beautiful too. For each its time. Tonight I saw a movie about enslavement and imprisonment. It touched me deeply and made me reflect on my own life. It made me realize that sometimes it is in the most gruesome times you find life's true beauty."

Once I was back in Austin I was officially on leave of absence, which meant I would not receive any income until I decided to go back to work. I did keep my benefits, so that was good. Because I wanted to stay put and did not desire to travel every week again as a consultant, I had contacted my former employer, Tivoli, and they were happy to talk to me. They could use an experienced SAP consultant, and I had been invited for an interview. The interview went well as far as I was

---

19.   Dr. Joseph Gold is director of the Syracuse Cancer Research Institute.

20.   Hydrazine sulfate is a nontoxic therapy that fights cachexia, a wasting syndrome that causes weakness and a loss of weight, fat, and muscle, from a disease such as cancer. Ross Pelton, RPh, PhD, and Lee Overholser, PhD, *Alternatives in Cancer Therapy: The Complete Guide to Alternative Treatments* (New York: Fireside, 1994).

concerned. It did not sound as though a lot had changed since I had left the company, except that they were still dealing with the same issues. I was not sure whether they were going to make me an offer. I just had to wait and see.

Benjamin kept up with his IVs and went to visit Dr. Rizov at the Austin Rejuvenation Center almost daily. In mid-December he had another blood test done and got the results back. The tumor markers had gone back up to 4,000! I did not understand. For some reason the Laetrile did not seem to work anymore. To think they had gone down 6,000 at a time while we were in New Jersey! And now they were going up.

Benjamin said he had known they would be up. Why was this? Did he feel it? Was he anticipating this outcome for some reason? The result kept him from continuing the IVs. Instead he continued with the B-17 pills and the apricot seeds. I had once again brought up surgery, and he told me flat out that the more I discussed surgery, the more he would go against it. He was still convinced he could beat this cancer with alternative medicine, doing it his way, or so I thought. I totally did not understand this young man. What could I do—how could I help Benjamin? I concluded that I was utterly helpless. All I could do was to contact Dr. Schachter for advice. I also contacted Dr. Contreras of the Oasis of Hope Hospital (Tijuana, Mexico) about Laetrile treatment. I contacted him to ask what these changes, up and down, in the tumor markers meant. Dr. Contreras, an expert on Laetrile treatment, had achieved quite some success with this therapy. Over the past six months I had several times suggested, unsuccessfully, to Benjamin that he go and receive medical care as an inpatient in Dr. Contreras' clinic in Mexico. I explained to Dr. Contreras that when we first went to New Jersey the tumor markers were as high as 21,900. Thanks to the Laetrile they went from:

- 21,900 to 16,000
- 16,000 to 12,000
- 12,000 to 6,400
- 6,400 to 858

and then started going up:

- from 858 to 1,100
- from 1,100 to 2,100
- from 2,100 to 4,000, all within a time period of six months.

Susan had talked to Benjamin on the phone a couple of times since he returned to Austin. He talked to her about his treatment options. He was thoroughly enthusiastic about Chinese herbs and Indian remedies and methodologies. Which was wonderful—if the results could be more positive, if he would combine them with some conventional treatments, such as surgery. But no one could talk him into something he was not willing to do. Susan again also strongly recommended the removal of the tumor in his testicle. He listened but did not make any promises. I had hoped that Susan could get through to him, because I as his mother could not. Susan and Benjamin had become very close during the months we lived up north. They had bonded, and Benjamin had confided in her. He told her things he would never tell his mother. But even Susan was not able to change his mind. It seemed nobody was able to change his mind. The helplessness was awful. There is nothing worse than watching your sick child when there is nothing you can do to make him feel better. That's where I was—feeling totally helpless. Until Benjamin changed his mind, I had no choice but to get on with my life ... to at least try to get on with my life. Christmas was coming up, and I needed to start getting ready for that.

Benjamin, meanwhile, started looking for apartments. He had enrolled in Austin Community College and was planning to start his studies in January. He found an apartment close to his college, in the center of town, and planned to move in mid-January. He told me he felt more comfortable by himself, that he could take better care by himself. However, I was not convinced. The way he was going now, he would not be able to look after himself at all. I saw a young man who was losing weight , who was constantly in pain—although he did not mention it to me—a young man who needed someone who was there to see to him on a daily basis. I still had not received a reply from either Dr. Schachter or Dr. Contreras about why the tumor markers had risen. I decided to request facts about surgery from the M. D. Anderson Center, hoping that by presenting him with written materials, with facts in a printed form, he might reconsider surgery.

In the meantime I had received word from Tivoli, my former employer, that I did not get the job. The guy told me that he really wanted me, but even with a considerable cut in salary I was still too expensive for him. Too bad. This meant that for the time being I needed to get back to the Information Management Group[21], as I needed an income, especially now that Benjamin was taking up his studies again and had his own apartment. He would need my financial support. In mid-December I received an answer to my e-mail to Dr. Schachter. He felt that Benjamin and I thought that if Benjamin received enough IVs he would be able to completely control the disease. Dr. Schachter did not think that at this point surgery would be helpful. It all depended on whether the cancer had spread to his lymph nodes and other areas. There were many additional things that could be done, but he pointed out that he could not even get Benjamin to agree to do the things he recommended when he sat in the room with him. So it was doubtful that he could be helpful now at a distance. He asked for a full list of exactly what Benjamin was doing and not doing. He was interested in the pathology report and any other lab work that had been done. He wondered what physician Benjamin was currently seeing and whether he was being regularly examined.

In my response to Dr. Schacter, I let him know the truth of the matter, which was that Benjamin was not seeing anyone. After the IVs seemed to have stopped working and the tumor markers had gone up again, he stopped treatments and saw no doctor. I was more than worried. Most of the time I felt sick to my stomach. I did not know what to do and how to persuade Benjamin to seek medical help.

Again I turned to the Internet, searching for answers, trying to find help and suggestions so that I could present them to Benjamin, hoping that he would run with them. I joined discussion forums, newsgroups, you name it—anything that gave me some sense of doing something. After asking people on the Internet about different therapies, one of the replies I received sounded very promising, an e-mail from a fifty-five-year-old gentleman that advised me to investigate ozone therapy. The gentleman was not a doctor, just a person who was interested in alternative medical procedures and in living longer and better. He told me that his business partner had developed prostate cancer a few years ago and had elected to do ozone therapy after refusing chemotherapy and the recommended surgery. His cancer, thanks to the ozone therapy, had completely gone, and he was now fine. In addition, this gentleman

---

21.   IMG is the company I worked for as an SAP consultant.

claimed that he had met many cancer patients once designated as terminal who were now fine due to ozone therapy.

I had never heard of ozone therapy before, but thanks to this e-mail I planned to research it and present my finding to Benjamin. The need to do something was unmistakable, as Benjamin was not looking good. As soon as he stopped receiving the IVs, his color had gone. He looked pale and was in pain most of the time. The painkillers weren't strong enough anymore. I did not understand why he did not do everything in his power to get rid of this disease. He kept buying alternative tinctures[22], but it was obvious he was not taking any of them—all the bottles were still unopened.

I e-mailed Susan almost daily, and she responded almost daily. She was just as frustrated and felt just as helpless as I did. She was suggesting that he go to the M. D. Anderson Cancer Hospital—not for surgery, but for a total analysis. Even if he would not accept their advice, perhaps getting a total assessment would help him understand his situation and maybe open the door to other treatment options. Even though Benjamin had totally refused traditional treatment and therapies, we never understood why he had not pursued a total and complete diagnosis from the top of his head to his toes. We were both very upset with Benjamin for being so stubborn. He thought he knew it all. For the life of us we did not get it. We did not understand this young man, who was highly intelligent but refused anything and everything we suggested. The more any of us attempted to push him toward something, the more he pulled in the opposite direction.

Once again I had a conversation with Benjamin. I tried to listen to him without becoming upset. He was determined to treat his disease nonconventionally. I did not know any longer whether he was stupid or what. Benjamin had bought yet another book, this one by Dr. Hulda Clark, called *Cure of all Advanced Cancers*. She was convinced that parasites, bacteria, and viruses caused cancer. I was willing to read the book and spent an entire day doing so. She claimed that she had cured 96 percent of terminally ill cancer patients, that her method would get rid of all toxins and parasites. Her method would get your own immune

---

22.   Tinctures are liquid extracts used for a variety of health purposes. For example, Benjamin had astragalus, which is an herbal extract used to support the healthy function of the immune system.

system working correctly, which would then heal the body. The book contained tons of "true" stories. The problem was you had to do so much to make it work: things like removing piping from your kitchen, removing all your cleaning stuff, and other bizarre things. It sounded all so unreal. She said she could cure cancer in twenty-one days! Another thing Benjamin was suggesting was to look into was Rife Therapy. This therapy, which uses a Rife device, was being rediscovered after a cover-up during the 1930s.[23]

I did not know anymore. He seemed to run from one thing to another, without taking the path he should really have taken, which was getting proper medical advice and treatment from medical professionals. Although I still question conventional treatment, that was how I felt at the time. I believed in Dr. Schacter's professional advice and wished Benjamin would have followed through with it. But just as during the past six months, none of my concerns, suggestions, or pleas made any difference. Benjamin was going to do this his way—only his way.

I was willing to go along with Dr. Clark's therapy for three weeks, even though I was not confident it would be effective. If the tumors still hadn't shrunk, if the pain still had not gone, I would need to send him to a clinic, if I could get him to cooperate. I asked him to get a total medical checkup. A brand new MRI center had just opened in Austin, and I hoped Benjamin would consider going for a checkup at this center. I suggested that Dr. Rizov could write him a referral. Benjamin never did.

Just a couple of days before Christmas I received an answer from Dr. Contreras from the Hospital Oasis Clinic. He had looked into the medical details I had provided him, and he had taken the time to discuss my son's case with his medical staff. He had come to the conclusion that Benjamin had a testicular choriocarcinoma, which is the most aggressive of the testicle tumors. No known chemotherapy was useful. He informed me that Laetrile only helps temporarily. He did not recommend surgery at this stage, because the cancer had produced a large metastasis, a secondary tumor, in Benjamin's abdomen and had invaded his lymph system. The only thing that could help, according to

23.   Rife therapy may be the most suppressed medical approach of all times. Rife frequency therapy is a term for the use of ultrasound to kill germs. See www.rifetechnology.com

Dr. Contreras, was a combination of radiation therapy and the complete Oasis program, although his chances were very slim. He ended his message by saying that Benjamin's survival was going to be very short.

The message scared the hell out of me. My heart sank to my stomach. I could not believe what I was reading. It was all a nightmare. From the beginning I was convinced that Benjamin would survive this disease and that he would live. Or had I been in denial all this time, refusing to see the consequences? I had read so much on testicular cancer on the Internet; even the American Cancer Testicular Web page suggested strong survival rates, even at stage four. However, the treatment option was always conventional, meaning chemotherapy, and Benjamin would never agree to that. It had to be his way. He could not be persuaded to go the conventional way. He just did not want to hear. I was beginning to think there really was another reason for his refusals, though I had no idea what it was. But his behavior was not normal, and I could not understand it. I was scared and felt hopeless and helpless. Benjamin was unique, and he had chosen to live his life this way. It just broke my heart to think of the consequences if none of the treatment options worked. I loved him dearly, and all I could do was to support him the best I could and go along with his choices.

On Christmas Eve Susan called me on the phone. She had been informed via e-mail how Benjamin was doing, because she wanted to be kept updated now that we no longer lived in New Jersey. I had forwarded Dr. Contreras' findings, and she was shocked. She tried to cheer me up and to make everything better. Of course she could not. All I was doing was hanging in there, trying to stay full of hope and trying to celebrate the holiday season as if everything were okay. Susan knew how much time I spent searching for answers and therapies and participating in discussion forums. She hoped that I would find the right combination of treatments and increase Benjamin's odds to improve the quality of his life. Her wish for the coming New Year was for Benjamin to get well, to be able to get on with his life and fulfill all of his dreams. That's all I wished for Benjamin myself, and I made a commitment to myself to do anything in my power to help him to get well.

Just before the year ended I contacted Saul, the ozone therapy guru. He lived in Canada and had a degree in chiropathy. I forwarded him the e-mail I received earlier that month that referred me to him. I had explored his Web page and had seen several methods described. And I asked him what type of ozone therapy would be best for Benjamin. All of the methods involved using ozone, which is composed of three oxygen atoms, to kill cancer cells. Within a day he replied and commended Benjamin for his good choice of refusing chemo, radiation, and surgery, which do not support the immune system. The only way to clear cancer from the body permanently was through the immune system, according to him. The best protocol would be the ozone steam sauna. Supposedly there were two clinics in the Austin area that were offering this protocol. I could not reach either of them and wondered whether I could purchase the ozone steam cabin myself so that Benjamin could treat himself at home. Saul offered both the ozone generator and steam cabinet for sale. He explained it was extremely easy to operate and anyone could learn it in ten minutes by following the instructions.

I discussed the ozone therapy with Benjamin, and he was enthusiastic about it. We thought it would be a good idea and much easier if he had his own set. I decided I would purchase the generator and the cabin. Saul informed me that there was a rental cabin being returned soon and that I would be able to purchase that from him for a reduced price. He suggested I contact a doctor in Maryland who's ozone generator was for sale. She could no longer use the generator because apparently ozone therapy was not allowed in Maryland, and therefore she was breaking the law. The authorities had threatened to close her practice if she did not stop offering ozone therapy to her patients. She whispered on the phone when I contacted her, so afraid someone would overhear the discussion and inform the authorities. It was sad, really, that in the United States, Land of the Free, you were not free to make medical care choices and that there was no room for alternative therapies. Too many doctors had been prosecuted and had their practices raided by the authorities.

While I was in the middle of getting more familiar with ozone therapy, reading up on it on the Internet and finding discussion groups related to ozone therapy, I had a very nice surprise: a surprise Mike had been able to keep a secret, as he knew that Zoë had made arrangements to come and visit. Just a couple of nights before New Year's Eve, early in the evening, the doorbell rang. Mike insisted I go to the door to see who it was. I opened the front door, and there stood my daughter Zoë and her boyfriend Frido. It was so very good to see them and so totally unexpected. Frido had left the choice up to Zoë whether to go on holiday to some nice resort somewhere in Europe or to come and see her mom, and of course her brother, during the holiday season. She had chosen the latter. Their visit brought a nice break from worrying about cancer, from doing more research, gathering more information.

We decided the celebrate New Year's Eve Dutch-style. That meant we prepared *oliebollen*—similar to donuts but round, with raisins, only eaten on New Year's Eve and the first couple of days of the New Year; *bitterballen,* a savory snack eaten with a bit of mustard, and *slaatje,* a traditional Dutch potato salad. I enjoyed preparing these Dutch goodies together with my daughter. It was fun.

Ken, Mike's son, who now lived by himself, had come down to celebrate New Year's Eve with us. It had been a long time since we all had been together, and we enjoyed each other without worrying too much. It did not last long though, because before we knew it their visit was up and I had to drop them off at the airport. I remember standing at the airport staring into the sky long after their plane had taken off, tears rolling over my cheeks. It was not fair; it was not fair at all. Why did my son have to have this disease, why couldn't he be healthy like most young man his age?

Benjamin was preparing to move into his own apartment, which he had rented from mid-January. I was not convinced this was the right thing to do, but I let him go regardless. I realized that he wanted to move on and to live a normal life without being reminded of his disease constantly. Going back to school meant a lot to him. He was in good spirits. Benjamin was so enthusiastic about the ozone therapy that while we were waiting for the arrival of the ozone generator and cabin, he decided to start another type of ozone therapy at Dr. Rizov's practice. Rizov administered this therapy by drawing blood, ozonating it, and placing the blood back into his body. This ozone therapy was called autothemotherapy. Benjamin would receive this therapy twice a week.

In the meantime I had tons of questions for Saul. What else did we need apart from the cabin and the generator? Would he need additional nutrition, pills? Would he need other type of ozone treatment once we had the sauna? Saul reassured us that once Benjamin was using the ozone steam sauna, it would not be necessary to have other treatments. He also informed us that ozone saunas were superior to autothemotherapy in efficacy for cancer.

I had met a professor online who was all for ozone therapy. Professor Campbell of the Integrative Medicine University of Technology resided in Australia and was very willing to share his findings. He found that a combination of alternative and traditional treatments produced the best outcome for cancer patients. He recommended a chemo based on cell culture together with the alternative treatments we now had in place. Apparently, in California there was a lab that was having great success with selecting chemotherapy based on culturing the tumor cells from a biopsy. It made sense to me, but persuading Benjamin to go for chemotherapy was another topic.

I had been on leave of absence since the previous November; it was now January 2000. My money was beginning to run out, and I needed to start thinking about a job. Because my job application at Tivoli had not worked out, I was considering picking up my consultancy work again. IMG had called and wondered whether I was willing to go to Europe for a couple of weeks to perform testing on the latest version of the SAP IS-AFS module[24].

What's more, Benjamin's lawyer had been in contact. While we were in New Jersey, we never heard from him, but the case was still open, and during the past six months nothing serious seemed to have been done about this, apart from some plea-bargaining back and forth between Benjamin's lawyer and the prosecutor. His lawyer wanted Benjamin to plea guilty to another misdemeanor so that he could keep him out of jail. Benjamin adamantly refused to do so. It made no sense to plead guilty to something he never did. Benjamin was not guilty of anything. That souvenir knife from Spain in the back of his car was just unfortunate. He wanted a fair trial so that he could defend himself and prove his innocence. Apparently America's way of dealing with justice was very different from the one in the Netherlands. I just did not

---

24.   IS-AFS stands for Industry Solution Apparel and Footwear Solution. It is SAP's ERP solution for the apparel and footwear industries.

understand it all. The only thing I did comprehend was that Benjamin could end up in prison. I decided to call his lawyer and find out more about it. His lawyer suggested not to try the case but to plead guilty and go for an informal program, which meant community service and probation. Benjamin was in no condition to do community service. He was in pain almost 24/7. Most of the time he needed to lie down to feel somewhat comfortable. There was nothing for me to do but to send the lawyer Dr. Contreras' e-mail to show the seriousness of Benjamin's condition. I suggested that I could pay an extra fine or fee to reduce the probation and community service. I begged the lawyer not to let Benjamin know I had contacted him, because I knew he did not want me to interfere with this.

Benjamin had moved out mid-January, was living by himself, and had started school. His apartment looked nice. He put up curtains and made an effort to make it look like home. It was small, with a small living room with just enough room for his sofa and bookshelf; a small bedroom, which he used for a study; and a small loft, walk-in closet, bathroom, and kitchen. I guess it was fine for a student.

The sauna steam cabin was expected to arrive shortly. The ozone generator itself had already arrived. Benjamin would be able to take daily ozone steam saunas in his apartment. There'd be no need to pay for expensive autothemotherapy anymore and no need for him to go out every other day or so to go to Dr. Rizov's clinic. The sauna would help him in several ways, destroying the cancer cells, detoxifying his system, and helping his lymph system. I was worried about going to Europe and staying away for two and a half weeks, but I realized I needed to move on. I felt it was now all up to Benjamin. I had handed him the tools, found holistic doctors, and made suggestions. It was up to him to use it all and do what he thought was best. He wanted to be self-sufficient and independent; I just prayed to God that he would follow through and get better.

Susan kept in contact with Benjamin and had spoken to him since he had moved into his apartment. They had talked about school and Benjamin's passion for writing, and also about his tendency to be "far out" in his thinking. He was happy and pleasant and had much to say; he wanted to talk. I dropped by almost daily to cook dinner for him and to see how he was doing. One day Benjamin returned early from school because he had been in pain and unable to sit up straight through his class. He was not very pleasant to me and wondered whether he could hang in much longer. I told him he had options as far as the pain was concerned and that he could have the tumor removed if he wanted to. But of course, as always, he said he would never have that done. So my last hope was that the ozone sauna would shrink the tumors and thus reduce the pain. Although he was in pain, he did not look too bad.

I finally received a copy of the letter from Dr. Khoory to Dr. John Garofalo, Benjamin's oncologist while we lived in New Jersey. I had been after this for quite some while, as it had never really been clear what the exact outcome of the biopsy had been. Here is what it said:

> A needle biopsy of the left supraclavicular region shows collection of what appears to be benign cells, and more significantly, tissue fluid was obtained with it. The above certainly does not look like embryonal cell carcinoma, however, the possibility of a teratomal element is certainly to be considered and hence the submission of this specimen to the hospital cytopathology.

> Thank you for the opportunity to evaluate this young lad; I will discuss the above with you as we obtain the further results mentioned.

I intended to call Dr. Garofalo to find out if the "specimen" was ever submitted to the hospital cytopathology and what the results were. When I did reach him, his response was vague, so I contacted Dr. Khoory about the outcome of the specimen submission, and his assistant referred me to Dr. Garofalo. However, Dr. Garafalo referred me back to Dr. Khoory, and I ended up with no answer. I wondered why they were saying two things. I gave Benjamin a copy of the report and urged him to see a doctor and have tests done; he would not have to do what they would tell him, but at least he would know where he stood. Maybe the tumors were all benign. I did not understand why he wanted to guess and worry all the time when a simple and painless test could give him peace of mind, no matter what the results were.

I traveled to Europe on Saturday, January 29, 2000. I would be in Germany for two weeks. I flew from Austin to Memphis to Boston to Amsterdam to Munich. It was an awful time of the year to do so much flying. I hoped that I would not get stuck anywhere because of snowstorms. I was scheduled to fly back to Philadelphia on February 13, 2000, and would stay over a couple of days to drop by the IMG office. If time permitted, I intended to drop by Susan's. I was very worried about leaving Benjamin, but I had to. I needed to pick up my life and start earning a living again. But that did not stop me continuing with my research about any and all cancer therapies out there.

I was in frequent contact with Saul because I had been reading lots of e-mails and articles about an oxygen therapy user group. I asked him whether injecting ozone into the tumor would work to shrink the tumors. Benjamin's tumors, the visible ones, were pretty large, and all the alternative treatments so far had not decreased their size. Another question I had was about the pain. Benjamin was in pain every single day and took painkillers, which he did not really wanted to do. But without them he was miserable. We were assuming that that pain was caused by the tumor mass in his lower abdomen. I was asking Saul all these questions because the doctors and oncologists did not know. All they suggested were surgery and chemo. They had not been able to answer our questions. Benjamin had now given up on doctors totally and refused to see any of them.

Susan had promised me to call Benjamin frequently during the weeks that I was in Europe. He needed someone to talk to, especially now that he was beginning to express his feelings of wanting to give up, whatever that meant.

Saul responded that it was not common to inject directly into tumors. If done, it was almost always into breast tumors, because there is no major artery to hit if the needle is off the mark. He suggested using a funnel over the tumors to concentrate the ozone there, which would have the same result and without the pain of the needles. The pain Benjamin felt was caused by the growth of the tumors pushing their way between the other cells. It would subside when the tumors stop growing. He recommended IP-6, a B vitamin derivative, which was useful for halting tumor growth. Toxins in the body were responsible for the tumors in the first place, and the removal of toxins in the ozone sauna would allow the body to clean up the tumors.

The sauna cabin arrived, and I was able to drop it off at Benjamin's apartment the day before I left for Europe. It gave me some peace of mind that Benjamin would be able to start a new therapy, which he could easily conduct himself without anyone's help, for the couple of weeks I would be gone. Using the sauna was simple; the person sits comfortably with the head exposed out through the top of the unit. A towel seals the opening around your neck. The ozone generator and the oxygen supply are then turned on, and the ozone is fed into the cabinet. The ozone is absorbed transdermally (through the skin), which is very effective at detoxifying the body and oxygenating it at the same time[25]. The oxygen is utilized by the body to remove wastes through enhanced blood circulation. Ozone also kills germs and bacteria on the skin. For tumors and such, a funnel (on a hose) can be attached to the inside of the outlet where the ozone enters on the inside of the cabinet, and this concentrates the ozone directly into the tumor itself. The sauna is portable and requires no plumbing. You simply plug it into the wall socket, fill the boiler with water, and turn it on. The action of the steam sauna serves to heat up the body, thus producing hyperthermia, which is very effective at stimulating the immune system. Elevating body temperature alone can destroy bacteria and viruses, get the lymphatic system moving, and increase the metabolic rate of the organs in the body.

While in Europe I had a chance to visit with my daughter, relatives, and friends. It was good to be away for a while. I actually took some time to have a good time. Benjamin was on my mind, though, every single day, and I was still very much worried about him. I went out for dinner with friends and Zoë. I even visited my ex, Benjamin's father, while in Holland. Wayne had just moved into a brand new three-bedroom townhouse with a very large loft.

During my visit to Holland, a friend at the time introduced me to a Reiki master. Zoë and I visited him, and he claimed he could

25.   Ed McCabe, *Flood Your Body with Oxygen: Therapy for Our Polluted World*, 6th ed. (Miami Shores: Energy Publications, 2003).

relieve Benjamin of his pain at a distance, using energy. He said it would take him four to six weeks to get rid of the pain. He also, after looking at Benjamin's picture, told us that Benjamin would not die from this disease, that he would get better again. He also mentioned that Benjamin was very angry with his father. I was willing to believe anything and was willing to pay for distance pain relief therapy. I welcomed anything that would give me hope, that gave a sense (even if it proved later to be false) that things would work out okay and Benjamin would get better. Looking back now, this was of course total nonsense. He was just another person who was trying to make a buck out of someone who was desperate, and I was fool enough to want to believe all this.

I arrived back in Austin around the third week of February 2000. The first thing I did, of course, was visit Benjamin. He was glad to see me. The previous night he had written in his journal: "I will see mother again tomorrow. Over two weeks it has been now. Funny, how I feel now compared to two weeks ago. One difference is that two weeks ago I wasn't sure I would see mother again, or should I say she me, alive?" I felt bad that I had been out of the country and that I had not been there when he turned twenty-two on February 2—again I had missed his birthday. I spoke to Benjamin about the Reiki master, what he had said about him getting well, about his anger toward his father.

I had hoped that Benjamin would have been well into the ozone therapy and that he would have used it every single day since I had delivered it to him. However, the opposite was true. He had barely used it, and I felt disappointed. The sauna had been sitting there for three weeks, hardly used. When I questioned Benjamin about it, he said it did not feel comfortable because the steam came from the pipes at the bottom, and the steam was very hot against his legs. The same thing was true for the steam coming from the pipes against his back. Again I contacted Saul, who instructed us to use rolled-up towels to prevent the steam from blowing directly on Benjamin's legs and to prevent it from coming up the back and being too hot. Very few people ever said they did not enjoy the sauna, Saul assured me.

It was obvious that Benjamin, once again, had not followed through with either his promises to me or with his therapies. I was not only disappointed but also very worried. He did not look good. He had not been to school, as he could not make it through class because of the constant pain. I now know I had been far too hard on him. I had no idea about the pain he was suffering, which paralyzed him and made him incapable of doing things. Not until later when I found his writing did I find out. Benjamin wrote: "Physical pain. My will seems too weak to equal it. I don't know how much longer I can take this. When will I break? Have I already reached a point of no return? Or would that point be death? Am I really as content with dying as I think? Or is there more for me to do? And how will I know? Death must be a breeze compared to the suffering of life. Oh, my pain. How long is it humanly possible to bear? Finding that out would certainly kill me. Is that what I want?"

Then out of the blue Benjamin mentioned that he was considering returning to Holland. I wondered what brought that to mind. When he was first diagnosed with cancer, I asked him whether he would not prefer to go back to Holland, but he had rejected that idea. He had said that if he were to die of the disease he wanted to die here in Texas, and he wanted his ashes to be scattered over the hills around Austin.

A couple of evenings later he called me on the phone in tears. He was crying and in terrible pain. I asked him if he wanted me to come over, but he said that it was not necessary. Then something went wrong and we were disconnected. I returned the call, but he wanted me to get off the phone. A minute or so later he called me back again, and he told me that he was very angry with me, that I did not love him, that I did not care. I felt hurt, told him he should go back to his father, and hung up. I called Wayne and asked him to call Benjamin and talk to him. It was obvious that he needed someone to at least listen to him, to comfort him. But it was not me he wanted to talk to right now. No matter what I said or did, I could not do any good in his eyes, or so I felt. Anything I suggested was ridiculous or nonsense. He seemed to know it all. I just wished that he would come and live with me so that I could be there for him and take proper care of him, but he refused. He did not want to be with me and Mike, under one roof—and that was where the problem was, why he would not live with me.

The next couple of days Benjamin changed his mind about whether he wanted to go back to Holland or not. One day it was yes, the next day no. But finally he made up his mind and decided to go back. I felt it was a good idea for him to go back. His father was living by himself.

He had just moved into a brand-new home with plenty of bedrooms, and he was not working. He was home all day long. In my eyes he had all the time in the world to look after Benjamin. I knew Wayne was on welfare and that he did not have much income, but I was willing to give him a monthly fee to take care of Benjamin, and I would give Benjamin a monthly allowance so that he would not have to ask his father for money.

Benjamin said that he wanted to return to Holland as soon as possible. Therefore I needed to start making arrangements right away. I was able to book a flight for him to leave Houston on March 4, 2000. Benjamin needed proper painkillers so that he would be able to persevere through the nine-hour flight. I booked a business class ticket for him so he would have a bit more leg room and a more comfortable seat, hoping the trip would be more relaxed for him. There were also tons of arrangements to be made on the other end. Although Wayne had just moved in to this new townhouse, it had barely any furniture or carpets. Adjustments needed to be made to what would be Benjamin's room, up in the loft. Zoë promised she would help Wayne and buy whatever needed to be bought. I would reimburse them for all the extra costs. I e-mailed Wayne and Zoë almost daily, letting them know what I wanted them to do and supplying them with all the relevant information about Benjamin. It was important that Benjamin treat his disease seriously now and that he really would try to get better. I had strong hope that with Wayne on top of him that that would happen. Benjamin was worried about the fact that he was not a Dutch citizen, partly because he might be disqualified from receiving national health care, but also because the Dutch government could deport him if he did not have a job.

In 1978, the year Benjamin was born, an old law still applied in the Netherlands: a baby born in Holland would automatically receive the nationality of its father, regardless. Wayne was British, so both Zoë and Benjamin automatically at birth received the British nationality. Zoë had her nationality changed before she turned twenty-one. Benjamin had omitted to do so before he left for the United States in 1996. Now he felt he did not really have a country to call home. He did not really have a home in Holland, nor in England, nor in the United States.

He really wanted to belong, wanted to belong somewhere, and that somewhere was now Holland.

When he returned to Holland, he needed to be registered at the local town hall. He also would need to apply for national health insurance. I was hoping that he would trust the doctors in Holland and that he would be very, very serious about his treatments. I advised Wayne to pressure Benjamin about having the testicle tumor removed. Benjamin himself seemed far more worried about the tumor in his neck than in the testicle. I was not that concerned about the neck tumor. I believed that that tumor was not cancerous. I expressed my feelings; I was enormously worried about Benjamin. He was far too thin, and he was in pain all the time. I said that I hoped Wayne could get things done that I could not. Because it was obvious we could not carry on like this any longer. It was time for real action.

In addition to making all sorts of arrangements for Benjamin, I also needed to ship his belongings. I wanted to ship his ozone generator and his sauna, but before I could do so, I had to return the generator to Saul, as it needed to be converted to 220 volts. The next thing was to contact a doctor who could prescribe stronger painkillers. The Vicodin tablets Dr. Rizov prescribed were not strong enough; neither were the Vioxx pills. Neither really worked for Benjamin. I decided to ask Dr. Schachter for a prescription, but Dr. Schachter did not feel comfortable doing so. He had not seen Benjamin for many, many months, and I was asking him to write a prescription for a controlled substance. He felt Benjamin's situation did not sound good, and he did not want to be part of encouraging him not to see a physician before a prescription is written. Dr. Rizov was not licensed to write stronger prescriptions. The only thing I could do was to make an appointment with an oncologist here in Austin, something Benjamin had not wanted me to do so in the past. However, this time I decided not to ask Benjamin but to just go ahead and do it. I would just make an appointment and take Benjamin along. The appointment was scheduled for February 28, just a couple of days before he would leave for Holland. The doctor could then examine him and perhaps give him the medication Benjamin needed.

Amazingly Benjamin did not protest and went along to the appointment. I stayed in the waiting room while Benjamin was visiting with the oncologist. The man appeared to be quite nice, and Benjamin liked him. He urged Benjamin to consider chemotherapy. He claimed that with chemo he would be pain-free within two weeks and better in twelve. Benjamin had advanced cancer, and his survival rate was 85 percent. The oncologist said it looked as though the cancer was in his lymphatic system, and it needed to be cleared out. It did not look like it had spread to his vital organs. The doctor even called a young man who also had testicular cancer and was now on chemo. Benjamin spoke to this young man on the phone. But neither of them could convince Benjamin to stay for chemotherapy. Benjamin decided to return to the Netherlands. Fortunately, the oncologist prescribed him stronger painkillers to enable him to fly across the ocean without too much pain.

Susan communicated with me through e-mail almost daily. She and Benjamin had bonded in a special way, and she cared about him very much. Susan worried about Benjamin and was a bit skeptical about him going back to live with his father. She was not so sure Wayne would be able to do a good job taking care of him. She wanted to know whether Benjamin had told me what treatment, if any, he would be pursuing in Holland. Of course he had not. He did mention however, thermotherapy and that he needed a physiotherapist to help get his strength back. He also wanted a trampoline to stimulate his lymph system. She wanted to hear something little more constructive, different, something other than this. She wondered whether he had a plan. It was hard on her—she did not understand his patience. I tried to convince her by letting her know that I was shipping all his stuff, including the ozone generator and sauna, which he had not been using so far, hoping that Wayne could persuade him to do the saunas, something I had not been able to do, no matter how hard I tried, how much I begged and pleaded. I knew if Benjamin did not take some serious action once back in the Netherlands, he would die.

Susan had talked to Benjamin on the phone. They had gotten into a heated discussion about discipline. She mentioned he lacked discipline, that this was causing him not to pursue proper treatment. Benjamin took her remarks as an insult, and he became defensive. All she was doing was to try to find out why he did not complete what he started. She said it was like having a conversation with the Wayne of old, who never accepted being told what to do and seemed to enjoy being contrary. During this conversation with Susan, Benjamin was being very protective of Wayne. She just hoped that they would be able to communicate and get things done. Benjamin wanted to reconcile with his father. She understood that. She asked Benjamin about his future; he said silly things about a short life. Then he sugarcoated it with positive words. He told her that the Hyman name ended with him. When he realized what he had said, he tried to cover it up. She wanted to know why he was like he was. Did he want to live? He was unique, and very special. He had the power and control to kick this disease; why did not he? She felt so hopeless—she needed to understand and she did not. She was grasping at straws to understand what made him tick. Benjamin was too intelligent not to know what he was doing and why.

Not just Susan, but I, his mother, also did not really know what made him tick. Benjamin had always kept very much to himself. He had never genuinely shared his thoughts, dreams, and concerns with me. Only in the past couple of years had I begun to get to know him a bit better, because he finally opened up to me and began to tell me how he felt. He was very, very spiritual, and I was very down to earth, which did not make it easy for me to understand his way of thinking. I knew he was very sensitive—something I was not. I did enjoy his company tremendously, and I was very proud of my handsome son. I loved him dearly.

I forwarded tons of e-mails to Wayne from doctors, vitamin companies, people who had given me advice—basically any communication I had that would help him get caught up with Benjamin's situation. I asked him to begin to start setting up appointments with doctors—not to ask Benjamin but to just do it and take him. I also felt he should have another biopsy to identify exactly what the cells were that were mentioned in the biopsy report. It was not clear whether the tumor in his neck was cancerous or benign. However, it was obvious something needed to be done about it. His lymph nodes needed to be clean, since this is one of the first places cancer usually spreads to.

There was a nontoxic alternative on the market called 714X[26]. 714X alters the consistency of the lymphatic fluid, enhancing the lymphatic system's ability to remove toxins from the body. The 714X needed to be injected daily in the right groin area. The *48 Hours* news program had a segment featuring people with serious cancers who had full remission using 714X. And of course the famous Billy Best[27] used this therapy for his cancer treatment after he refused chemotherapy, and Billy Best was fully cured. The difference was that Billy Best followed his regiment around the clock and was totally dedicated for six months. Benjamin was very wishy-washy, starting one thing, then another, and never following through. That was the most frustrating part. I did not have a problem with him choosing the alternative route; I had supported him in his choice. I just could not understand his patience, as Susan called it. I could not understand how he could just try one thing just for a couple of days and move to the next. Did not he realize that if he didn't treat this disease seriously he would die? Why was he gambling with his life?

Wayne e-mailed me, informing me that he was going to be very serious about getting Benjamin well again. He was looking forward to him coming over. He said he was going to make this his life goal, his number one priority. In the meantime, Zoë was making sure that Wayne's house was in order, that Benjamin's bedroom would be comfortable. A new laminate floor had been put in, a new bed and wardrobe had been purchased. Wayne had started to search the Internet himself and was receiving e-mails from all sorts of people who were willing to help and let us know their findings. I was pleased that he was being proactive. In a few days, Benjamin would fly out to Holland.

We had been shopping; he needed a few things, such as new shoes, some comfortable clothes for the plane, and additional natural remedies. We did not last very long shopping, because Benjamin could barely walk for longer than half an hour without pain and getting very tired.

---

26.   714X is a nontoxic health product, designed by Gaston Naessens, biologist, to enhance natural defenses and the immune system. Pelton, *Alternatives in Cancer Therapy.*

27.   Billy Best made the national news in 1994. He was on chemotherapy but ran away from home to get away from the chemo. He left his parents a note explaining that he felt the chemo was killing him rather than curing him. He was cured using 714X and Essiac tea. See also www.billybest.net/

I talked to him and once again stressed the fact that he now needed to get very serious and take large steps toward getting better; if he did not he would die. He realized all that and he wanted a personal trainer, someone who could help him to build up his muscle mass once he was back in Holland.

Apart from that he wanted someone who could direct him medically, someone he could trust. I had been searching online for him and found several people in the Netherlands who could fulfill that role. All this information I e-mailed to Wayne, hoping he would act on it and contact these people. Benjamin mentioned to me that he was finally considering having his testicle tumor removed. Therefore I asked Wayne to enroll Benjamin immediately in the Dutch national health system. I would copy all the medical records and details I had and make sure Benjamin had the papers with him when he left.

Friday, March 3, was the day before Benjamin would fly. I talked to Susan on the phone to let her know the latest. I would pick Benjamin up the next day at 10:00 AM, and we would drive to Houston. It would take us three hours, but I had a mattress in the back of my Jeep to that he could lie down if he wanted to when he became to tired to sit. He was really looking forward going back to Holland again. I hoped he was going to take his treatment seriously from now on. Wayne had already scheduled a couple of appointments. I had been talking to Wayne almost daily, as there were lots of things that needed to be done.

Zoë had been pretty busy helping out also. She had been cleaning the house, buying stuff. She had been at her father's all day that day. Sarah, Benjamin's little half-sister, who was just four, was there also. Her mother had left her with Wayne for the next couple of weeks. I thought it would be nice for Benjamin that everyone was going to be there when he arrived. I was glad that Wayne would be there with him all day. I had hated Benjamin living by himself for the past couple of months because he really needed constant help. Klaas was also going to meet him at the airport when he arrived. I just was hopeful that all of them would help to make sure he stuck to his treatments, whatever the treatments were going to be. So yes, in a way, I was glad that he was going back to his father. He would be surrounded by family and friends who loved and cared about him. I needed to let go; besides, I needed to get back to work and pick up my life where I had left off ten months ago.

Mike and Ken came down to Benjamin's apartment in the center of Austin to say good-bye to him. We were ready to get in the car and drive to Houston's International Airport for his flight back to Amsterdam. There were no direct flights from Austin, but there were from Houston. Rather than taking a local flight to Houston, we thought it would be best if we drove down, even though it was a three-hour drive. At least we would have some extra time together, and I would be there to help him in Houston. Benjamin would not have to walk from one terminal to another. It would have been too much for him.

The trip itself went fairly well. Benjamin was able to withstand the three-hour drive without too much discomfort. I was worried about the nine-hour flight though. Once we arrived at the airport, it seemed to take forever before it was time to board. I could see Benjamin was getting extremely tired, and sitting in the uncomfortable airport chairs did not help. Finally, the passengers were allowed to board, first and business classes first, which included Benjamin. I wished him success and expressed my desire to see him healthy the next time I saw him. I hugged him, held him close, and told him I loved him. I waited until it had taken off and stared at the plane. I wondered how many times I had stood there, either picking someone up or seeing someone off. And how many times had I left and come back? So many tears had been shed here. I was sad. My heart ached, and I felt the pain.

CHAPTER 5

Holland

Hey Mom, I am dying
Why aren't you here?
Hey Mom, I am crying
Don't you want me to be near?
                    Benjamin Hyman, Spring 2000

Benjamin arrived back in Amsterdam on Sunday morning, March 5, at 8:15 AM. His father, both sisters, and his best friend, with his girlfriend, were there to meet him. They went back to Wayne's house and celebrated his homecoming awhile. Benjamin made the trip okay—he had survived. I received an e-mail, midmorning my time, from Wayne that Benjamin was okay, that he was now sound asleep, and that Benjamin probably would give me a call when he awoke.

After Benjamin had left there were still tons of things for me to arrange. I needed to take care of his apartment and his bills, such as the telephone and utilities. I called the lease office and explained what had happened and why we had to break the lease. I promised I would pay the rent for the next coming month and empty and clean the apartment until it was spic and span.

The ozone generator had been shipped back to Saul to be converted to 220 volts, and I was waiting for it to return so that I could ship it, together with the sauna, to Holland. I had made arrangements for a shipping company to collect all Benjamin's possessions on Tuesday, March 7, but I was not going to make the deadline. The generator was not back yet, and I had to fly to Pennsylvania to work on March 7 through Friday, March 10. The shipment had to wait until I returned and so was rescheduled for Monday, March 13. It was going to be shipped by air freight and would be delivered at Wayne's front door within the following couple of days. It was important the shipment arrived as quickly as possible, because apart from Benjamin's belongings, it also contained all of his herbs, vitamins, and medications. He needed those as soon as possible. Sea freight would take weeks, if not months.

I e-mailed Wayne that I had gone through all Benjamin's papers, and I would send them via overnight air. These papers included the original protocol Dr. Schachter had prescribed. I noticed several recommendations, such as hydrogen peroxide IVs, large doses of intravenous vitamin C together with Laetrile, tons of vitamins and minerals, plus a special diet: protocols we had not been very familiar with last year when we first visited Dr. Schachter. Looking back, it seemed a very good protocol. It was just a big shame that Benjamin at the time had decided not to accept many of his recommendations and just stuck with Laetrile.

On Sunday, March 19, I spoke to Benjamin on the phone. He told me that he was not feeling well at all. I began to worry again, especially because he was not doing anything then. How could he? The sauna had not yet arrived. I suggested to Wayne that he made sure he ate the apricot seeds daily and drank diluted hydrogen peroxide[28]. I ordered hydrazine sulfate, which I had direct shipped to Baarn. Hydrazine sulfate helped starve the cancer and increased the appetite, helped with weight gain, and increased energy; it even helped with pain control. I hoped that this time Benjamin would take these pills. Several doctors, including Dr. Schacter, had recommended hydrazine sulfate.

I e-mailed both Wayne and Zoë on a daily basis. I told them what Benjamin should drink, what he should eat. I forwarded them all my

---

28.   Hydrogen peroxide is a molecule of water with an extra atom of oxygen attached. Because the ozone steam sauna had not yet arrived, drinking hydrogen peroxide could be an alternative.

research results. I probably overloaded them with information. I just could not just sit and wait. I felt I needed to stay involved. I did not only research American Web sites but also the Dutch ones. I found and ordered interesting vitamins and health products I thought could be beneficial. I also researched Web sites for different hospitals to see what type of therapies they were offering, where they were located, what they were doing for testicular cancer. I searched for orthomolecular doctors, naturopaths—any specialty that I thought could be of help. Would Benjamin be interested now that he was in Holland? Would he perhaps take more action now that he was being looked after and cared for on a daily basis?

I e-mailed my mother, brothers, and sisters to let them know that Benjamin had returned to Holland and that he was living with his father. I mentioned that we felt it was better this way, as Wayne had all the time in the world to look after him, while I had to work. Wayne would be taking care of him physically; I would be taking care of him financially. I informed them that I was back at work since the beginning of March and I expected to start working on a project sometime in April or May in Connecticut for six to eight months. I would then come to visit every month, as flying from New York was much quicker than flying from Houston. However, it was not yet set in stone; I would know more soon.

Benjamin received the 714X from Canada but was hesitant to use it because several lymph nodes were very large. He could feel several of them in his body; some of them were visible, like the one in his neck, which now was the size of an egg. We still were not sure whether these enlarged lymphs were cancerous. He was afraid that if he used the 714X it would upset whatever was in his lymph and cause severe toxification. He would consider it under supervision of a doctor. His fears were ungrounded because 714X is totally nontoxic and could not hurt him. It is designed to open up the lymph and boost natural defenses and the immune system.

I started looking for a doctor in the Netherlands who would be willing and able to help Benjamin with the 714X. I thought I found a young doctor who actually had been to the United States and knew Dr. Schachter. This young doctor was very impressed by Dr. Schachter but did not believe in 714X. He argued that the medical community did not write about it, and he felt Dr. Atkins promoted this product too much. He believed the product was too commercial. So much for that ...

In the meantime, I continued e-mailing user groups. Over the months, I had made contact with various people who were also working with alternative therapies. Ozone therapy came up several times, and one man, Dr. Stephen Duncan[29], had been very successful with ozone therapy. He had treated three cases of advanced lung cancer in the past five months. All cases had been cleared. He did a combination of cupping over the tumors in the sauna and cupping over the tumors lying on a table. The hyperthermia sessions lasted thirty-five minutes, and the cupping sessions were forty-five minutes. He administered two sessions a day, five days a week, for four weeks. In two cases all tumors disappeared and the lungs were on the mend. The third case was the most severe; the lady he was treating had seven tumors in her lungs. One was reported as grapefruit-size, and the other as baseball-size. Five of the tumors had completely disappeared, and the remaining two were about quarter-size. Each patient drank a liter of ozonated water after each session.[30] He advised me to start Benjamin on ozone therapy right away.

Benjamin had been back in Holland a couple of weeks. In mid-March I forwarded mail I was still receiving at my address in Austin to Benjamin at his father's address. I decided to include a letter. Perhaps written words might make more of an impression than talking on the phone. The letter was dated March 16, 2000.

My dear Benjamin,

First of all I want you to know that I love you very much. I miss you, and you are on my mind every single day. Secondly, here is some mail for you that has arrived here, including your international driving license. By the time this letter arrives, hopefully all your stuff that I

---

29.   Dr. Duncan is a licensed massage therapist, Reiki master, certified hyperthermic ozone therapist, licensed holistic health care practitioner, and energy worker, practicing in the Dallas area.
30.   The author received the detailed medical information about these patients originally from discussion groups on the Internet. It was subsequently confirmed by Dr. Duncan.

shipped has arrived. I also hope that you started using the ozone steam sauna and that you really are very seriously doing everything possible to get well. Benjamin, I am at a total loss! It breaks my heart to see your health deteriorate so much—from a healthy young man to a young man who can barely do anything … a young man who, if he does not do something soon, will be dead within the next year! How can I say that? Because I do not see you getting better. Since last year May your health has gone downhill bit by bit.

Every day I ask myself over and over again, why you are not using all the stuff you have available, such as Essiac tea, Laetrile, apricot seeds, the ozone sauna, etc. etc., on a daily basis. You yourself decided to choose alternative therapies. All of us have supported you in that decision—we have offered you all the tools. I can't do it for you, Benjamin. Only you yourself can take the pills, can sit in the sauna. You cut yourself short by not being consistent. As a result, you are now almost unable to do anything. Why didn't you grab all the opportunities offered? I can think of a couple of reasons:

You don't have the discipline and are afraid to ask for help; or you just don't want to get better, because now everybody is paying attention to you. If that is the case, it is the wrong attention. Or you really are afraid and you stick your head in the sand, as you don't want to know. Maybe the reason is none of the above. I may never find out, and therefore I may never understand. If you don't have the discipline to do what needs to be done on a daily basis, please let people around you help you. Ask them for help! If you don't, you are only punishing yourself. Whenever you want to visit a doctor, say so right away; don't wait until a week has passed. People would only be too happy to help you, but you will need to ask them. Just put yourself in their shoes. You would be only too happy to help if people asked for help. In retrospect I blame myself that I did not take firm action. I should just have dragged you to doctors and specialists. But then again, knowing you, I wonder whether that would have done any good. I still can't forget what you said last year when that one Dutch boy was dying of cancer: "We cannot just let him die." But I should just let you die? I hope you realize that you need to take on all the possibilities—and that now you need to really take action. I hope that you take the hydrazine sulfate and are considering the 714X therapy. I hope that you have yourself examined medically, that you will let professionals guide you.

You have several options:
- Don't do anything—we all know the end result of that.
- Choose the conventional option—chemo, surgery, etc.
- Choose alternative therapies and then commit fully, 100 percent.
- Choose a combination of conventional and alternative.

Who cares what method will heal you, as long as you get better? That's what we all want—your father, Zoë, I, Susan, Klaas, etc, etc. You need to make a choice and commit 100 percent. Don't just try one thing then switch to another, but grab all options and stick to it. Just letting you know that I ordered Ellagic Red 21 pills for you. Ellagic acid pills are from red raspberries and prevent destruction of the P-53 gene by cancer cells. Also I printed some information about a Japanese mushroom, the coriolus versicolor, that is supposedly a cancer inhibitor. Zoë told me she found a physiotherapist for you, but you'll first need a doctor's referral.

Well, Benjamin, I am going to print this letter and mail it. I hope you will read the entire letter, that you'll make the right decision, and that you'll follow through.

I love you,
Mother

Exactly two weeks after Benjamin returned to Holland I called Zoë and learned that both her father and Benjamin were visiting. I spoke to Benjamin, asking how he was, and he expressed his desire to be admitted to a clinic, not a hospital. Had he already received and read my letter? I wondered. He was looking for a clinic that could guide him and help him to get better again; he expressed his desire to work with a physiotherapist. He talked about water therapy, steam therapy, thermotherapy. I was not sure whether there were clinics in Holland that offered those kinds of therapies. Benjamin complained about the pain he was suffering. He had not felt well at all that day, and he had taken a bath at Zoë's, which made him feel a bit better. Wayne had only a shower in his bathroom, no tub. Benjamin claimed the painkillers the Dutch doctor had prescribed did not work. He barely slept, he said, and was awake most of the night.

I asked Rob, the Reiki master Zoë and I had visited in February, for his help. As a Reiki master, part of the alternative circuit, surely he would be able to advise me. I asked him about the painkillers and whether there was a possibility he could get the ones the Austin oncologist had prescribed. I asked him if he could help to find clinics that would offer the therapies Benjamin was looking for. Rob did try to offer some help, but he was not able to get the same painkillers, and, in the end, his search for alternative clinics was not successful.

I was beginning to get worried. I realized that it had only been two weeks since Benjamin left, but I could not help feeling that things were not going the way I had anticipated. Things between Wayne and Benjamin did not work out as well as I had hoped; they ended up arguing quite a bit. Perhaps, I thought, I should ask my sister-in-law if she would be willing to look after Benjamin. Mike said I should let it be and give Wayne a proper chance. He was taking action, maybe not as aggressively as I would have liked, but he was trying. He was working on Benjamin's national health insurance, and he was talking to the local government in Baarn about Benjamin's nationality. He had made appointments, and Benjamin was scheduled to see an oncologist in the VU hospital in Amsterdam on Friday, March 24.

Susan contacted me by e-mail, wondering how Benjamin was doing with his father. I mentioned that I spoke to them on the phone regularly and that Benjamin was staying with Zoë over the weekend. He had finally begun to realize he needed help and needed to do everything he could to get better. I told her that he was scheduled to see a cancer specialist in one of the best hospitals in Holland; this doctor was doing gene research for cancer and he had been on TV just recently. In the meantime, I wrote, I was searching for a clinic because he was in pain every day. I told her that he had lots of support in the Netherlands. Klaas and his girlfriend came by regularly. My family was willing to help him, both financially, if needed, and otherwise. I mentioned to her that I was back at work, working from home, but there was a possibility that I would be working in Connecticut from the end of April until the end of the year. If it all worked out, I had told my manager that I'd rather they rented an apartment for me in Connecticut as opposed to flying me back and forth to Texas each weekend. I would prefer to fly to Holland once a month to see Benjamin. But we did not have the project yet. We had worked on the proposal, and now we just had to wait and see.

I contacted Stephen, the gentleman who had been so successful with the ozone therapy, because I had several questions. Besides Stephen, I contacted Saul again. I asked both of them whether they knew of any clinics in Europe that could treat patients with ozone therapy and the other therapies Benjamin had mentioned. I hoped that Benjamin would start using the ozone steam sauna as soon as it arrived in Holland. Rob, the Reiki guy, had informed me that there were no alternative therapy clinics in the Netherlands, but that there were in Germany. He found a couple, and he had scheduled an appointment at a clinic in Sunden on April 11. He let me know that he was willing to go to the clinic with Wayne and/or Zoë and Benjamin. The clinic worked with thermo water therapies and ozone therapy. That was good news. I continued searching the Internet for clinics in Germany and was amazed that there were so many different options. Most of them sounded wonderful, and it gave me hope.

Benjamin called me a couple of days later. He was still staying at Zoë's. It was five o'clock in the morning his time when he called. He told me he wanted to be admitted to a clinic as soon as possible. He did not want to just go for an appointment but wanted to stay. I was worried about this call. What did it mean? Was his health deteriorating rapidly? Or was he trying to run away from the appointment with the oncologist at the VU hospital? Benjamin had called because he felt things had become yet more critical. In his journals at this time, he wrote, "I have been here three weeks, almost three weeks. It seems like every time I pretend to choose life, life says bad choice." I was also worried because he had not started any therapy since he arrived.

His sauna had not yet arrived. I was very disappointed with the service of the shipping company I had shipped eight boxes by air from Houston to Amsterdam and had requested and paid for three-day service. The goods had arrived in Amsterdam on March 15 but had not been delivered to Wayne's address more than a week later. I contacted the shipping company and explained that my son was terminally ill and needed the goods in this shipment urgently. It was stuck in Customs. I received a reply from the Dutch Logistics Company explaining why it had taken so long and that it would be delivered as soon as it had been cleared.

The day Benjamin visited the oncologist in the VU Hospital, he called me to let me know the results. The oncologist had wanted to admit him to the hospital and to treat him with chemotherapy. Again Benjamin could not be convinced, and he refused the doctor's treatment. In the meantime Rob had been able to reschedule the appointment at the German clinic. It was now set for Monday, March 27, rather than April 11. Benjamin wanted Rob to accompany him. Another appointment with a different clinic was scheduled for April 3.

I called Benjamin after they went to Germany to learn the outcome of their trip. Once again he was staying with Zoë, not his father. Questioning him about it, I discovered that things were not working out too well between them. Benjamin said he was staying where the atmosphere was positive, and that was at Zoë's. He and his dad could not have a nice relationship because Wayne did not have a nice relationship with himself. There seemed to be some kind of confrontation going on between the two of them. I needed to talk to Wayne to see what was going on. Wayne could be very defensive, obstinate, and difficult. It could be hard to get through to him.

In the meantime I was searching for a clinic again. The visit to the clinic in Sunden, Germany, did not work out. The clinic had expected Benjamin to do conventional treatment first. After that experience, Benjamin cancelled his other appointment with the clinic in Meschede. Saul and Stephen recommended we contact Dr. Kief in Germany, who worked with ozone therapy and was supposedly the best. However, this doctor did not have a clinic and only treated outpatients. This was not an option for Benjamin because he was a five hours drive away. I also e-mailed Mark Lester, who ran a clinic in London for outpatients and with whom I had communicated via e-mail in the past. Mark used ozone therapy, among others. I asked him whether he knew of any clinics in England and/or Europe where Benjamin could stay for three or four weeks to get the treatment he needed.

Then I came across a Web site about a clinic in Denmark: the Humlegaarden Clinic. It sounded perfect. Treatments included hyperthermia, light therapy, ozone treatment, orthomolecular treatments, and others. This clinic was one of the most well-known private clinics in Scandinavia that specialized in alternative or unconventional methods. It was exactly what Benjamin had been looking for. Diet was also important, and at Humlegaarden they served only vegetarian meals, based on a mixture of raw and cooked vegetables, legumes, cereals, fruit, and herbal teas. When we visited Dr. Schachter's clinic, we had been made aware of how important a healthy diet is. In his clinic we had received a long list of what foods to avoid and what to eat instead.

I contacted the clinic right away, explained that my twenty-two-year-old son had advanced testicular cancer and that he had received no conventional treatment. I asked them questions about whether the clinic would be able to treat him. Would he be able to check into the clinic within a week? Was staff available and would they work with the patient on an individual basis? I questioned them about their ozone therapy; did they have ozone steam saunas?

I forwarded all the information I found on the Internet about this clinic, hoping that Benjamin would be enthusiastic and go for it. I spoke to Benjamin on the phone as often as I could. In the beginning he gave me the impression that he really wanted to go to this clinic in Denmark. Then he changed his mind and said he wanted to go to London as an outpatient. He was still changing his mind all the time, still not wanting to make a commitment.

During one call, he did not sound well; he was in pain and uncomfortable. I could tell it was wearing him out to the point that all he wanted was to die. He just wanted to be taken to a peaceful place and die, somewhere in a forest where he could hear the birds sing, he had said.

I was beginning to panic. I could not get through to him over the phone, no matter what I said. What could I do? I e-mailed Benjamin, proposing that he choose a clinic of his liking to go and stay for three or four weeks for treatment and to gain some strength back. Then he could choose an outpatient clinic for follow-up treatments, perhaps the

Finchley Clinic in London. I wrote, "As soon as you have chosen the clinic, you surrender fully and cooperate totally. Trust the people that are treating you." I told him he had nothing to lose, that doing nothing would definitely kill him. He would die. I assured him that treatment in a clinic could perhaps help, could perhaps cure him. He could get better. I asked him why people like his friend Kathleen from Austin, the mayor of Austin, and Lance Armstrong—all cancer survivors—were still alive. Was it because they did not trust doctors, because the doctors wanted them dead?

I wanted to know why he didn't grab the chances that were being offered. How far did I have to go? Or did he want me to simply say: okay, Benjamin, just go ahead and die. Is that what he wanted to hear? I said, "If so, go ahead and find your place in the forest to die, but don't ask me to be part of it. A year ago when another young man your age was dying of cancer, you said we needed to do something. We could not just sit there and let him die. Your words! Should I now just sit here and let you die? What are you afraid of? Please answer my questions. I beg you, please explain so that at least I can try to understand. Tell me why people who did seek medical assistance and did receive treatment are crazy and you are not? They are perfectly healthy! And you?"

I also had another question for him: Why did he take painkillers, which were manufactured by the pharmaceutical industry? Why? Those medicines were pure toxins. Why did he not use natural remedies? Because in his case they did not work anymore! Why not grab any method that could make him better? Or would he rather die? I forwarded him en e-mail from Professor Campbell, who informed me that there were times when traditional medicine saved life. I did not know what to do anymore.

I was becoming depressed about the whole situation; it was a never-ending story. My entire life was centered around this awful disease, cancer. I went to bed and got up with cancer on my mind. It was all Mike and I talked about. It controlled my life. I communicated my frustrations to Susan; I told her that I had recently spent almost an entire day on the phone with Benjamin, trying to make him see that he needed to take action and do something. Every time came another excuse, as he ran from one thing to another. I did not know what to do anymore. Living with his father had made no difference whatsoever.

No one seemed to be able to make him change his mind and take some action. He was not doing anything as far as I knew, not taking pills, supplements—nothing, just the painkillers.

Susan suggested that I might be able to appeal to Benjamin's inner spirit. According to her Benjamin was behaving like a pure, true fatalist, believing that events are predetermined by fate and cannot be altered. But in actuality fate can be altered by free choice, by our spirit, which might then alter his visions of doom. Benjamin had the power—he could change his destiny, and by doing so, that would become his new fate.

I had forwarded her details about the clinic in Denmark, and she felt it was perfect. It seemed to offer all the options Benjamin would accept. She liked the fact that they also offered psychotherapy. With Benjamin that was so important. He needed to overcome his negative attitude and his anger, or whatever it was that stopped him from accepting medical treatment. Mike and I had even been talking about taking legal action. I was not sure whether that was in option in Holland. I needed to talk to Wayne about it. But before I would consider doing so, I still had hope that he would agree to go to Denmark, especially because he himself had expressed the desire to be admitted to a clinic.

I sent another e-mail to Benjamin, letting him know that I loved him very much, that all I wanted for him was the best. I wrote that I wished that I could take the pain, the disease, away for him, that I was sorry I could not. All I could do was hand him the tools, research clinics, buy ozone generators, etc. Now that he was in Holland, I asked myself whether I should just leave everything and go to Holland as well. I wrote, "I have come to the conclusion that that did not make any sense. It would not be beneficial for me unless you really would work hard to get well. If that would mean both conventional and alternative treatments, so be it. If that meant staying in a clinic, fine. If that meant being admitted into a hospital, fine also. Only then would it make sense for me to come to Holland—not as long as you are at Zoë's or your father's and you are not doing anything. In that situation I cannot add any value." Should I have felt guilty being here? Sometimes I did. But then I realized it did not make any difference where I was—not until Benjamin took action. Not until he told us what he wanted, so that Zoë, his father, and I could take action.

Regardless of whether Benjamin decided to go to the clinic in Denmark or not, I had in the meantime both spoken and e-mailed Dr. Andersen, the owner of the holistic clinic. I let him know I had discussed his clinic with Benjamin and that he was checking out his Web page. I wanted to know about the procedure to check into the clinic. Could Benjamin travel to Copenhagen the following Saturday, April 8? What did he need to bring? How were we going to handle the financials? I mentioned that my daughter most likely would take Benjamin to the clinic. Was it possible for her to stay overnight?

In the interim I also e-mailed all my Dutch relatives. I e-mailed them out of desperation and informed them that I no longer knew what to do with Benjamin. He was slowly but surely dying. I explained that I did not understand why Benjamin did not want any medical assistance. I told them I had found a perfect clinic for him in Denmark, where he could follow all his alternative therapies. But for one reason or another, Benjamin always had another excuse not to do it. I let them know that he was now permanently staying with his sister Zoë, as he and his father did not get along at all. Zoë took loving care of him, but I felt it was a burden for her, which she should not have to carry. I explained that just recently I had been on the phone with Benjamin almost an entire day, but it was impossible to talk sense into him. I was at a loss and could not think why he would not make a decision or do something about his health. What was he clinging on to? What did not he want to let go? What was he afraid of, in God's name? Couldn't we all together try to convince him that he needed to go to this clinic? Should we just force him and take him there against his will? Or should we just let him be and let him die? I did not know anymore. I could not carry on anymore.

Susan tried to call, but she could not get a hold of me. She realized that I had probably been on the computer and the phone all day, so she e-mailed me instead. She was curious if Benjamin had made a decision yet. I informed her that I had decided to go ahead and book Benjamin into the clinic regardless of whether he liked it or not. Wayne had made a commitment to take care of him, but instead Zoë, who had a full-time job, was burdened by the task. She should not have to do this. I figured once Benjamin went to the clinic, Wayne needed to be the one to take care of him and make sure Benjamin would stick to it. I expressed my concerns to Susan and that it was obvious something was terribly wrong with Benjamin. It seemed as if he was totally paralyzed or totally crazy. I could no longer let this rule my life. He was going to get treatment and get it over and done with. I would call Wayne and tell him that Benjamin was now going to follow our method, and he was going to listen. If we did not, Benjamin would continue destroying himself completely. I did not understand why, but I was not going to be part of it.

Then, on the last day of March 2000, I received an e-mail from Benjamin.

Mother,

Last night I had been thinking for a while. And believe it or not, the future for a change was looking beautiful. I had the desire to becoming healthy again; I had the desire to live. This is how it looked in my mind:

Monday I would go and visit Finchley's Clinic in London for a week. Daily ozone and Rife treatments and from there I'd go to Denmark. Work intensively with the different treatments (first agree with you and the doctor which treatments I will follow and which I won't) for three weeks, maybe two times for three weeks, so that I got well again and had my full strength back again. I'd change my lifestyle 180 degrees so that the cancer would not return. And then, after I have this behind me and I am a 1,000 percent better again, life after the treatments would look beautiful. I'd go to Australia for a period of time, work on a farm; learn how to become an organic farmer and take classes in school. In short, a total new start of something.

But the truth is, this is a fantasy far away from reality. I see the reality and that reality is totally different. I come back to the place where for me things are so bad. And I am afraid to fall back in the same rut and to pick up my old routine. I deserve a better life. The past years have not been easy for me, and it seems there is no end in sight. I don't want to be in pain my entire life. Not physically or mentally. I do have lots more to say but at the moment it is not coming out the way I want it. So, until next time,

Your son

I answered that, yes, he deserved a better life, without pain. I told him he could have that by working seriously on his health, together with people who cared for him. I said he needed to go to the clinic, to surrender and to accept help. I wished him a so-much-better life.

I asked myself why he had to suffer so much; what was the meaning of all of this? He never did anything wrong, never mistreated anybody; he was a kind young man, very spiritual, and he believed in the good of mankind. Oh God, how can I help him? I prayed. I wished I could take his pain away. My heart ached for him. I was so helpless, incapable of making him well. The only thing I could do was to have him admitted, even if that meant doing so against his will. I decided that was what I was going to do. I would, with help of my family in the Netherlands, force him to be admitted into a clinic or hospital.

Susan applauded my decision. She recognized that it was not going to be easy and that it would take a combined effort to pull it off. Benjamin should not have to live each day in pain, not when help was right around the corner.

Forcing him was not necessary, because in the beginning of April 2000, Benjamin agreed he would go to the clinic in Humlegaarden, Denmark. He would be treated in the clinic for three weeks. Zoë made flight arrangements for the both of them. They were flying Saturday, April 8, arriving at Copenhagen airport at 11:40 AM. Wayne was going as well, but he would drive by car. Benjamin realized this was his last chance, but he told Zoë he would refuse chemotherapy. He would not go near a place where they treated patients with chemo. This clinic did not do chemo if the patient did not want to; all the other clinics I had checked all offered a combination of chemo and alternative therapies. I intended to visit Benjamin when he was there, but I could not yet make any plans, as I was waiting to hear from my manager about my assignment to this project in Connecticut. I did not know when I was expected to be up there, but once I knew, I would be able to make arrangement to visit Benjamin in Denmark.

I spoke to Benjamin a couple of days before his departure for Denmark. He was feeling a bit better. He had moved back in with Wayne again and started arranging his room. However, while we were on the phone he was trying to find excuses for not going to Denmark. I then began to realize that he was extremely frightened—he was terrified. I had not realized before that he was so scared. I had asked him several times in the past whether he was scared, but he had always denied it. I reassured him that his father or Zoë could stay with him if that made him feel better but that he needed to go. It was important that he got medical attention as soon as possible.

It was time to inform my relatives, both in Holland and in the United States, that Benjamin was going to be admitted. My ex-family-in-law especially needed to know. I had not been in touch with Benjamin's grandma recently, and I was sure she was anxiously waiting to hear how Benjamin was doing. I received e-mails from Paula and Susan. They all were very happy to hear that Benjamin was finally being admitted to get the care he needed. They felt their prayers had been answered; they hoped and prayed that from here on, Benjamin would improve a bit each day. I had to promise to keep them updated on how he was doing.

Sunday morning I called Zoë on her cell phone. They had arrived in the clinic the day before. Benjamin was sleeping when I called, and she and her father were touring the place. Dr. Andersen himself had just returned from the United States, and they hadn't had a chance to meet and talk to him. I called again later that day and spoke to both Benjamin and Zoë. Benjamin had not said much, but Zoë sounded positive. They had seen the doctor, who had given Benjamin some shots immediately. They got on well with the doctor. He was nice, had a good sense of humor, and took action right away with Benjamin. The following day Benjamin was booked to go to the hospital, which was just down the road from the clinic, for x-rays and blood tests. Benjamin had been up all day, something he had not been able to do for quite some time. He had been eating all the vegetarian food and eating well, according to Zoë. When I called he was in the middle of putting a jigsaw puzzle together. So it all sounded positive. He seemed to have settled and decided to go for it.

They had befriended an American guy called Steve, who was there with his father, who had lung cancer. They had been there ten days, and the father was already off the morphine. It all sounded encouraging, and I was hopeful the treatment would do Benjamin good. I intended to visit Easter weekend. For now I let them be. I thought it would not be a good idea to call them daily.

Zoë returned home a few days later, and I spoke to her on the phone. She said Benjamin had a couple of tests back: his liver was okay, his immune system was low, his lymphs needed detoxifying. I intended to call Benjamin again the following Sunday when Zoë would be there again to visit.

I was still working from home. My main task was training a junior associate and creating end user documentation for the company in Connecticut. We did get the project, and so I would be going up to Connecticut, but I did not know yet when. I was first to go to Phoenix, Arizona, for approximately three to four weeks and then, most likely to Connecticut for six months. I was expected to start on April 24 in Phoenix. Because I was going to be in Connecticut for six to nine months, we thought it would be best if Mike moved there with me and we put our house up for rent. I contacted a realtor I had dealt with in the past and asked him whether there was a demand for corporate furnished houses in Austin. If so, how would we go about renting the place out?

During that same period I tried to contact Dutch Immigration and Naturalization Services. I was trying to find out what needed to be done to get Dutch nationality for Benjamin. Things would be so much easier if he were Dutch. He would be able to get national health care and qualify for welfare. I explained to immigration that I was Dutch, that Benjamin had been born in the Netherlands, and that he was raised as a normal Dutch citizen. But because of a silly, very old law, he had received British nationality rather than Dutch, even though he had never ever lived in Great Britain.

Once I knew what my next assignments as a consultant was and when I had to start, I was able to plan a visit to see Benjamin in Denmark. I scheduled my flight to Copenhagen, Denmark. I tried to call Benjamin, but for some reason I could never get through. Instead I wrote the clinic an e-mail and asked them to print the message and hand it to my son. I let Benjamin know what my plans were and what time I was arriving. I asked him how he was doing and said that I felt I had not talked to him in ages. If there was anything in particular that he wanted me to bring, let me know. I missed him and loved him and I would see him soon.

I left Austin on Wednesday, April 19, and arrived in Copenhagen on Thursday, April 20. I stayed just a couple of days, because the following week I was expected to be in Phoenix.

My visit with Benjamin was very nice. It was good to see him again. I had missed him. He looked reasonably well and he was doing okay. Not great, just okay. I was not sure whether his stay in Denmark had done him an awful lot of good, except that he got into the routine of eating regularly and getting the medical attention he needed. He was using mistletoe, doing hyperthermia treatment, and taking vitamin and mineral supplements for his treatment during this time. Dr. Anderson had tried hard to convince Benjamin to go for chemotherapy, which of course he refused.

The doctor was very pleased to see me. He thought that I would be able to persuade Benjamin. All I could tell him was that I had been trying for the past year but so far had not been successful. I again suggested to Benjamin that he undergo a combination of both chemo and alternative treatments. According to Dr. Anderson, he still had a very high chance of survival, between 90 and 95 percent, and testicular cancer was highly curable with chemo. I was hoping that Benjamin was thinking about it, but I was not at all sure about that. Now that he again had some blood tests done, we found out that his tumor markers were way up there again, where they were last year, at 22,000. His organs, including his kidneys and liver, were still okay. He did have large tumors in his abdomen and that very big tumor in his neck. According to the doctor, all these tumors would disappear if he did chemo. He would not need surgery, just the chemo. According to Dr. Anderson only three chemo sessions would be necessary.

The food in the clinic was excellent: completely organic and only vegetarian. The dishes that were prepared with just vegetables and whole foods were unbelievable. I spent some quality time with Benjamin; we enjoyed each other's company, walked along the beach, and just relaxed most of the time. We did talk about his next steps, and he still expressed the desire to go to London, to Mark Lester's clinic. The days flew by, and before I knew it I was back in a plane again. I had to change planes in Amsterdam and therefore had about half an hour to see my daughter Zoë. We had made arrangements to meet at the central meeting point. It was brief, but at least I got to see her before I left Europe again.

Upon my return home, I immediately contacted Mark Lester and informed him that Benjamin was currently at the Humlegaarden clinic. I told him that they had advised Benjamin to take chemo, which of course he had refused, but it was obvious that he needed to do something fast. If not chemo, he really needed to be dedicated to following a strict protocol, using the tools he had. Benjamin wanted to see Mark for a couple of days, as he felt he could learn from him what to do with the ozone steam sauna and the Rife device he had. The Rife device was another tool we had purchased while he was still living in the United States, but he had never really used it. I asked Mark if Benjamin could start his treatment at the London clinic and if so, when would Mark have time for him? How many days would he recommend Benjamin visit his clinic? After that he could continue the treatment at home.

I also e-mailed Benjamin that I had arrived safely in Austin and that I had e-mailed Mark Lester to ask him whether he thought it would be a good idea for Benjamin to visit Mark's clinic. Mark had replied, saying it would be an excellent idea. He could give Benjamin the right advice on the use of the Rife device and teach him how to self-treat with ozone therapy. He offered continued technical support afterward. He was also going to give him some electro-crystal therapy, which he had seen save lives in the case of prostate and bladder cancer, though he had not personally used it for testicular cancer. He recommended coming for three days and felt it would make a huge difference. He would have Benjamin for three hours a day and give him all three therapies: Rife, ozone, and electro-crystal. He also wanted to get him on some nutritional support. The clinic was very busy at the moment, but he would squeeze him in. There was a cheap local hotel nearby where he could stay if he needed accommodation.

Benjamin wanted to visit from May 3 to May 5. Unfortunately Mark was not sure whether he could get him in quite that fast. However, if he must come on those dates, Mark suggested Benjamin just turn up, and he would make sure he fitted in somewhere. There were always short-notice cancellations, so Benjamin would get fitted in, but he might have to wait a bit. In that case he would keep him busy reading what he considered to be essential material.

Benjamin returned from Denmark on Saturday, April 29, after three weeks at the clinic. Zoë went to pick him up, and together they flew back to Amsterdam. I was working remotely from home again. The trip to Phoenix had not materialized, which suited me perfectly. Benjamin was going to stay with Wayne again. I needed to talk to Wayne because I wanted to suggest that he allow Benjamin two to three weeks to work with the ozone very aggressively every day; if there was no change, we would force him to take chemo. I felt that the ozone therapy would help. Everything I could find on the Internet about ozone therapy was positive; besides, I had spoken to Stephen, who had successfully treated the lung cancer patients. At least it would give me peace of mind knowing that Benjamin was actually doing something on a daily basis.

Benjamin so far had never seriously used the sauna, except in Austin a couple of times for very short periods because he was uncomfortable in it. Again I forwarded an e-mail I had received earlier that year from Professor Campbell in Australia, who suggested both alternative and conventional therapies together, as that worked well. He himself worked with ozone therapy and found that ozone steam saunas had the best results.

The following day I spoke briefly to Susan, as it was her birthday. She had turned fifty-two. Susan and I were the same age, both born in 1948, and were very similar; we got on well together. I updated her on how Benjamin was doing, how he had experienced his stay in the clinic, and told her that he had a very high chance of being cured if only he would surrender to chemo. She could not understand why he still refused chemo. She could come to only one conclusion: that he did not want to live. Did he really not want to live? We discussed a strategy for assuring Benjamin that accepting chemo was not a sign of failure. Life is so precious, and we could not imagine anyone not wanting to enjoy the time they had on this earth. Benjamin was such a gifted person, so intelligent, and had so much to look forward to in life. Why did not he want to get better—or did he? Would we ever find out?

On Monday, May 1, Zoë e-mailed me to let me know that she had made all the necessary arrangements for Benjamin to go to London. She had ordered an airplane ticket, made hotel reservations, and booked a taxi to pick him up when he arrived. She had initially made arrangements for two people: for Benjamin and his father. But regretfully the two of them had been in a fight once again, and Benjamin would rather go by himself. He was scheduled to return the following Saturday. Benjamin was looking forward to going to London. Zoë had spoken to Mark on the phone, and to start with, Mark had freed up Wednesday morning just for Benjamin. She wanted me to respond quickly and to call her. I, however, had been spending time in airports all day long, as I was on my way to Baltimore. There had been a lot of thunderstorms in Texas, and many planes had been delayed. I finally made it in to my hotel. It was already 10:00 PM before I was able to e-mail Zoë and respond to her message.

I worried about the fact that Benjamin was going to visit London by himself. Was he capable of doing so? I wondered whether he was strong enough, whether he had enough energy, to do so. I was especially worried because he was no longer able to walk very far. I asked her whether she could not persuade Benjamin to have his father travel with him. They really needed to try harder to get along. Benjamin needed someone desperately, someone who could help and guide him on a daily basis and to make sure he stuck to this protocol. I explained that I was working in Baltimore the next couple of days and that I would be at the office in Kennett Square in Pennsylvania that coming Thursday. I would not be able to call her until then. I told her that I would e-mail Mark Lester to let him know I would send him a check for his services shortly.

I e-mailed Mark to let him know that my daughter had informed me that Benjamin would be seeing him that coming Wednesday. I was so glad. I let Mark know that Benjamin really needed to take dramatic steps, that he had wasted too much time, and that his health had deteriorated rapidly since he had finished with the Laetrile IVs. I also let Mark know that I had spoken to Stephen in Dallas and let Mark know which ozone protocol Stephen used and how successful he had been. So I had good hopes for the ozone.

Mark replied that he would like Benjamin to come in for three days, for four hours each day, and Mark would treat him with everything he had to offer: ECT, Rife, ozone, nutritional education. The purpose was to have Benjamin learn how to use the Rife machine and the ozone steam sauna most effectively, so that he could treat himself with those tools at home. After his visit to London, Benjamin would need to continue to use his Rife machine and give himself ozone seven days a week. Twice a day would even be better, but one would do. Long, aggressive ozone sessions worked best for cancer. Mark asked me for Steven's e-mail address or phone number, as he felt it was useful to communicate with colleagues.

On Wednesday, May 3, I e-mailed Zoë to let her know that I was back in Pennsylvania and that I would try to call her from the office the next day; if not I would call her Saturday from home in Austin. I was wondering whether she had already heard from Benjamin, had he arrived safely? The next day, Thursday, May 4, I received a couple of e-mails from Mark, telling me that he was doing his best for Benjamin and that there was a lot he could do himself with the equipment he had, but he also suggested a clinic in Mexico. He recommended that Benjamin should take hydrazine sulphate, as he was severely emaciated.

Later that same day I received a very worrying e-mail from Mark. Benjamin was supposed to have been in the clinic at 3:00 PM to continue his treatment, but by 5:15 he had still not turned up. Quite apart from the clinic time that had been set-aside for him, Mark was very worried about him, especially because Benjamin did not seem to have returned to the hotel. He asked me to phone him with any information I had about his whereabouts. But of course I had no knowledge of his whereabouts. I had not spoken to Benjamin that past week. Mark was going to call the police and would keep me informed. In a PS he informed me that he had telephoned the hotel, Zoë, the police and two local hospitals, which had made no admittance under his name.

Oh, my God, where could he be? I began to feel nauseated and was so very worried. I imagined him lying in an alley somewhere. What if he had been on his way to Mark's and his legs had given out on him? He had been complaining about one of his legs—what if he had fallen and was now lying somewhere to die? How the hell could Wayne have let him go by himself? This was ridiculous. Did not he have any sense? Wasn't his life goal to help Benjamin, to get him better? It had only been two months since Benjamin had returned to Holland; had Wayne already given up on trying to accomplish what he had set out to do? I should have believed Susan, who had questioned Wayne's capability from the start. I panicked. I did not know what to do. What could I do from 5,000-odd miles away?

Late that night I received another e-mail from Mark, letting me know that Benjamin was okay. Zoë had called and told him that he had checked into another hotel. But he was not exactly sure why Benjamin had not turned up or had not bothered to let him know. He was disappointed with Benjamin, because the previous day when he had turned up he was forty-five minutes late. Mark did not want to treat him any further because he did not work that way. But he was glad that Benjamin had been located and was safe. He felt this was one case where he just had to wish him well on his journey. He wrote that regretfully he did not feel Benjamin's omens were all that good unless Benjamin was prepared to work very hard. Benjamin came across as very intelligent, but too laid back about the whole thing.

I did not respond to Mark to explain exactly what had happened until the following Sunday, May 7. On Friday I had traveled back from Philadelphia to Austin but got stuck Friday night at the Houston airport due to thunderstorms and bad weather. I was forced to stay overnight in a hotel. In the meantime I had found out that Benjamin had been very ill and could not walk when he was in London. He had checked out of the hotel into another one, because the bed was so awful, it made his pain and discomfort even worse. He had wandered the streets in tears, trying to find another hotel that was more comfortable, taking just one step at a time and then resting; he had been exhausted. Finally he had been able to contact Zoë. Zoë had made arrangements immediately to get him out of there and had him flown back to Holland on the first available flight, which was a plane to Rotterdam rather than Amsterdam. She had to explain an awful lot to the staff at the London airport, because they were hesitant to let him leave due to the physical state he was in. Zoë and Frido had driven to Rotterdam to pick him up. The ground staff had put him in a wheelchair. But thank God, he was now back in Holland. The whole London event had been a drama, a nightmare. I felt totally helpless again. Here I was on the other side of the world, ten hours flying time away. What in God's name could I do? How could I convince my precious, beautiful son that he needed to get conventional treatment?

After a year of struggling and battling, I was beginning to lose all hope. Bills started to come in from different doctors, clinics, and Rob the Reiki guy. I questioned Dr. Anderson's bill, as it was not itemized, just a large sum. I wanted to know what I was paying for. I wanted to know whether Benjamin had received treatments the last week he had been in the clinic, because I got the impression from Benjamin that no further treatment was given after he had refused chemotherapy. If that had been the case I would be paying too much.

Everybody wanted money, and so far not very many had been able to do much for Benjamin. I began to see them as money grabbers. This Rob guy was a money grabber: how could I have been such a fool to believe that he could take Benjamin's pain away from a distance? Distance healing? Bullshit! That's what Dr. Anderson told me; nobody could heal the kind of pain Benjamin was experiencing from a distance. I had been a sucker; I had been taken advantage of by so-called holistic healers, by people who abuse desperate people who are willing to pay dearly for hope and promises. I was sick of it all. I asked Rob what his medical credentials were. Of course he did not have any. Why hadn't I asked him this upfront? Besides, weren't healers supposed to heal rather than charge outrageous fees like this Rob guy did? The world sucked and was getting more sick every day. They were all in it for the money. I felt a fool.

In desperation I wrote an e-mail to a therapist in Holland, a guy called Luuc whom Benjamin had seen a couple of years ago when he was suffering from extreme sweating that had caused Benjamin emotional stress. I knew Benjamin liked and trusted this guy. This past year I had suggested to Benjamin several times that he seek professional mental help, but without success. So I contacted Luuc to ask him if he would call Benjamin. I gave him Benjamin's cell phone number. Perhaps, so I hoped, Benjamin would open up to him and let him know why he was killing himself. Maybe he would be able to find out why Benjamin, in my eyes, was committing suicide. I had decided as of right then that

I was going to distance myself from Benjamin's illness, because after fighting for a year and trying to do everything possible for Benjamin and trying to understand him, I could no longer work up the energy. I needed to move on with my life. I should not let this disease control my life every single day. As a last effort to try to get through to Benjamin, I was e-mailing this therapist. Maybe he could find out what Benjamin's fear was, what kept him from wanting to get better. For some reason Benjamin did not trust the medical world and did not dare to surrender. It was incomprehensible why he wanted to suffer daily. Several doctors had told him he could be free of pain within a couple of weeks. He was hanging on to something, but what was it?

As much as I vowed to keep my promise to distance myself from Benjamin's illness, it wasn't much later that I realized that that would prove impossible for me. As I write this, eight years later, I can see that I was simply in no way capable of just letting go and distancing myself from Benjamin's disease. I could not change that dynamic, no matter how much it might have helped me at the time. Thoughts like *What kind of mother am I, residing thousands of miles away from him? I need to be close, I need to be nearby,* made me return to my former role soon after I had resolved to let go.

On my birthday, May 9, I received a telephone call from the American author Ralph Moss. Dr. Moss had written several books about cancer, including *Questioning Cancer Therapy* and *The Cancer Industry,* among others. Dr. Moss was visiting Dr. Anderson in Denmark, and Dr. Anderson had mentioned Benjamin's case. Dr. Moss called me to find out Benjamin's telephone number, as he wanted to talk to him to see if perhaps he could convince Benjamin to go for chemotherapy. In the end I don't think the two of them did get a hold of each other, due to phone problems. It was all so sad. That coming Sunday marked the year anniversary since Benjamin was diagnosed with cancer. As it was hard to get Benjamin on the phone these days, I decided to e-mail him one more time. The e-mail was dated Wednesday, May 10, 2000.

Hello, Benjamin,

Just imagine … that within four weeks or so you don't have any pain anymore

Just imagine … that your tumors disappear
Just imagine … that you sleep well again every night
Just imagine … that you feel well again
Just imagine … that you can do things again
Just imagine … that you have your energy back again

It can all come true …

Benjamin, I beg of you to consider all therapies … also chemo. If this, together with all alternative therapies, such as ozone, Essiac tea, you name it … can make you better, then please go for it. I can understand if you are scared. But nothing is worse than the pain, the stress, the misery you now have to go through. We are all here to support you, to help you overcome your fear … Do you remember what I said before you went to Denmark? "Right now you are not looking forward to it at all. It seems like a huge mountain you need to climb, but soon, once you have been that big mountain, you will look up and see, in retrospect, that it was only a very small mountain. It was not that bad after all." Wasn't it the same with the IVs? In the beginning you did not want to go to Dr. Rizov; looking back, it was not that bad. This is how it will be if you just surrender to your fear and grab with both hands all the therapies that are being offered. Let the medical world help you, before it is too late. If you wait too long the cancer will spread to your organs.

You still have a chance. What is more damaging, the chemotherapy or constantly swallowing drugs against the pain? The chemo is only for a couple of times. After that, you are through with it. Together with the ozone steam sauna, you will have killed the cancer cells in no time, and you, you will be on the road to recovery, to becoming healthy again. According to Dr. Anderson, and I can check this for you with Dr. Doty[31] if you want, a chemo cycle is just a couple of days of chemo, then nothing for three weeks, then a couple of days of chemo, then nothing again for three weeks. This is repeated three times. Besides the chemo, you can continue with the alternative therapies.

---

31.   The oncologist in Austin who prescribed the painkillers for Benjamin before he departed for Holland.

It is even better to do so, according to Professor Campbell[32]. A combination of conventional and alternative approaches saves lives. I think you should not think about it too much. Just do it … just surrender. Let go of whatever it is that is stopping you. If you are afraid talk about it with Zoë and the doctor or whoever, try talking about it with other fellow-sufferers. There is a contact group in Amsterdam of young men who also have testicular cancer, or who did have it.

Below this e-mail are two addresses and phone numbers for these groups. We are all there for you. Today I spoke to Zoë on the phone, and she said that you and she are working on a protocol and that you need daily help to follow through. Therefore, I have e-mailed your aunt Marianne and asked if she would be able to take you into her house and help you until I have taken care of business here so that I can come to Holland. Marianne does have the room to put you up. She has an extra bedroom with a connecting bathroom downstairs. You could have your own bed moved over there, together with the sauna. As you know, Ralph Moss called. He asked me to ask you to call him, but I understood from Zoë that that did not happen. He gave me his fax number. He also told me that testicular cancer is one of the few cancers that react very well indeed to chemo, as I said when I e-mailed you when you were in Humlegaerden. He also mentioned he had a new book out: *Antioxidants against Cancer*. The book reveals how you can use antioxidants to greatly decrease the side effects of chemotherapy and improve the results of chemotherapy. By the way, the Japanese mushroom also helps with the chemo.

Carolyn Myss, the author of *Anatomy of the Spirit: The Seven Stages of Power and Healing*, writes:

"Combine your internal healing with any conventional medical treatment that is essential, and stick to the program. Reach out for any support that you require, and use the support appropriately. Don't waste time by thinking, acting, or praying like a victim. Do all that is necessary to support your physical body, such as taking the appropriate medicine, eating properly. Simultaneously, do all that is necessary to support your energy body, such as releasing unfinished business and

---

32.   Professor Campbell, from Australia, fully believed in the power of ozone steam saunas. He treated all sorts of disease with the ozone saunas.

forgiving injuries from the past. Talking does not heal: taking action does. While it is essential to work at maintaining a positive attitude whatever your illness, healing requires dedication and commitment. Healing one's body or one's life challenges requires daily practice and attention. All circumstances can be changed in a moment, and all illness can be healed."

Tonight I have ordered caster oil for you. I have not ordered the Homozon yet. Castor oil is a laxative. Did you know that? Well, Benjamin, I am going to stop. It is bedtime for me. I have addressed this e-mail to both you and Zoë's addresses, as I am not sure whether you still use this address. I'll also print this and snail mail it to you, as Zoë mentioned that her printer was without ink.

I love you and I miss you.
Mother

As I was working from home again for a few days—the following week I would be in Phoenix all week—I had some time to e-mail Benjamin's relatives in the States. Paula was pleased to hear from me and appreciated that I kept her and her mom, Benjamin's grandmother, informed about how Benjamin was doing. It had been extremely hot in New Jersey for that time of the year, reaching over 90 degrees F—temperatures that were normal for Texas but not New Jersey. She was sorry to hear about Benjamin and had hoped that by now he would have changed his mind and listened to the doctor's recommendation. Paula had advocated for conventional therapy all along. When Benjamin was first diagnosed with cancer, she had done everything in her power trying to persuade Benjamin to go for chemotherapy. She had not been as open-minded about the alternative therapies as her sister Susan had been. Paula now realized that it was up to Benjamin and that none of us were able to make him do something against his will. She wanted to let me know that she thought about Benjamin many times each day and that we were both in her prayers. Mother's Day was coming up, and she wished me a nice Mother's Day.

Then I talked to Zoë on the phone later that afternoon, Friday, May 12, exactly one year after Benjamin had been diagnosed with cancer. I received the good news that Benjamin had finally decided to have himself admitted into a hospital. That was *great* news. I could not have thought of a better gift for Mother's Day. I was extremely happy and relieved. Zoë was going to make arrangements; Benjamin wanted to go that coming Monday. In the meantime I had purchased Ralph Moss's new book and ordered Japanese mushrooms and MGN3 for Benjamin. I had direct-shipped the goods to his father's address in Baarn. I also e-mailed my brother and sister to see if they could help me find a rental home. I had definitely made up my mind to return to Holland within the near future. Even though Benjamin was going to be admitted into a hospital, I did not stop wondering about lots of things. I e-mailed Dr. Andersen in Denmark and asked him about the chemo treatment. I wanted to know whether he was confident that Benjamin was going to be well. What would chemo do to his immune system? Why were Benjamin's legs so badly swollen? Was this lymph edema? If so, what could be done about it? I hoped he could give me the answers; any reassuring advice would be very much welcome. I informed him that I was traveling next week and would not be reachable by phone, but he could e-mail me.

And so he did. He reassured me that a certain protocol was followed in all Western countries and that the Dutch doctors knew all the details of this protocol. He was very confident that the treatment would be effective and that Benjamin would be completely cured. Regarding the swollen legs, he mentioned that when Benjamin was in Denmark they thought it was lymph edema, but Benjamin should be watched for the possible development of venous thrombosis.

I e-mailed Zoë to let her know that I was traveling again, in Phoenix, a nine-hour time difference from Holland, and would be difficult to get hold of by telephone. I let her know the hotel I was staying at. I asked her to let me know by e-mail how things were going. I told here I would try to call whenever possible and that I might do so from my client's office, but that I would converse in English rather than in Dutch. I did not want my client to know that I was calling internationally at their expense. But there was no other way, as in those days I did not yet have a cellular phone. I needed to stay in contact and needed to be kept up to date with what was going on with Benjamin. Over the following days I received Zoë's e-mails daily. On May 15 she wrote:

Dear Mama,

Don't think the best of the good news right away, but I picked up Benjamin after work, and we spoke in the car. He really wants to get well, and I assured that he was going to make it. I have asked him whether he would like to take a vacation in September, and he really wanted that and is looking forward to that. He promised he would take all his medication and that he will eat everything that is good for him, regardless whether it tastes awful. Dad was here at my place also. Benjamin wanted him to come. He took a bath and felt well. I have given him ozonated water a few times, and he did take all his pills, including the MGN3. I really want you to ask somebody whether he can take the hydrazine sulfate together with the painkillers—I am not sure whether that is allowed.

Dr. Paul Hoekstra (the psychiatrist) could not do much for him. He had a bit of a shock, I think, when he saw Benjamin. He did say that he would guide him mentally as soon as he is better physically. Tomorrow the family physician is visiting, and he will provide an urgent referral note (or whatever you call that). Dad called Dr. Gerritsen at the VU Hospital, but he was sick—just had an operation or something. Dad is going to call his assistant tomorrow to find out who else is good and available in the VU. Apart from that I can't say one way or another. Hopefully I'll know more tomorrow. Benjamin really needs to be admitted this week. Haven't spoken to my manager yet about days off or unpaid leave of absence, but I don't think it will be a problem. They are all behind me and very supportive. They are not going to be difficult, and if they are, too bad.

Good thing that you e-mailed Finn[33]. Did he respond? Benjamin is really going to make it! I am convinced! Soon we will all be going on a vacation together and celebrate that he is well again! Even if it costs ten million! You come back to Holland together with Mike and rent a house here. Mike has his pension, and you can go and teach, an ordinary normal income. Money won't be important soon, but if I win the ten million I would not mind either, LOL!

I am going to bed; it is already past 1:00 AM. I love you and miss you. I think of you the entire day.

---

33.   Finn is Dr. Andersen's first name.

Lots of love and hugs from me.

P.S. Of course I'll keep you updated.

I replied that I was glad that Benjamin wanted to get well again. I wished her lots of strength and hoped that Benjamin would be admitted very soon. I told her that I was working hard to find a way to return to Holland as soon as I could, but that I still did need to work for the time being, to make sure I was covered for health insurance. I kept stressing the fact that Benjamin needed to use the ozone sauna daily to help him detoxify. (In retrospect, I realize Benjamin was in no condition whatsoever to use the ozone sauna and sit in the cabin for thirty minutes daily.) I also looked back over the past year at what we had gone through with the original Laetrile therapy, which did work so well in the beginning. I began to think that the tumor markers had started rising again the end of last year due to not detoxifying. Everything went well until Benjamin got that tumor in his neck. That's when his immune system was going down, because his lymph system was not working optimally. I wondered whether the toxic waste got stuck in his lymph system. If we had paid attention to detoxifying and had made sure his body had gotten rid of the wastes, who knows? His markers might have gone to zero. Instead the lymph node in his neck had become bigger and bigger.

At that point in time, from reading Zoë's e-mails I had no idea how bad Benjamin's condition really was. It was not until later that Zoë told me that he was not able to walk. She had even gotten crutches for him. He had to drag himself up the stairs to get to the bathroom. When he took a bath Zoë had to be with him because he could not get in or out by himself. She stood crying when she noticed how awfully thin he was, nothing more than skin and bones. It was a miracle that he was still alive.

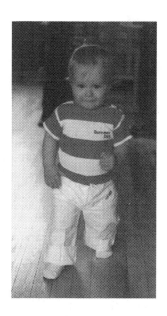

*Spring 1979. Benjamin just fifteen months old. He was a beautiful,
blond little guy and the sunshine of my life.*

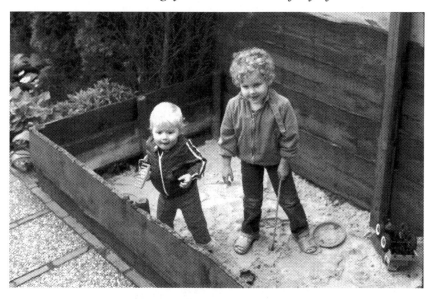

*May 1979. Together with Zoë playing in the sandbox. Zoë and Benjamin
were very close when they were little, but also during the rest of their years
growing up.*

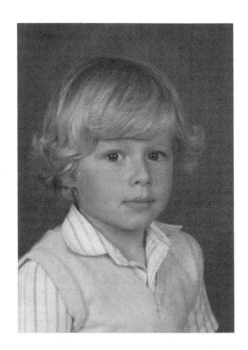

Benjamin's first school picture (kindergarten). School season 1982/83.

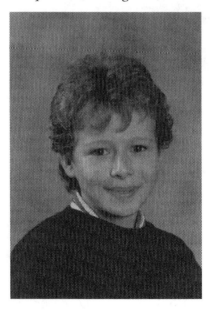

Elementary school picture. In this picture Benjamin is 8 years old.
Benjamin was very intelligent and his school results were always excellent.

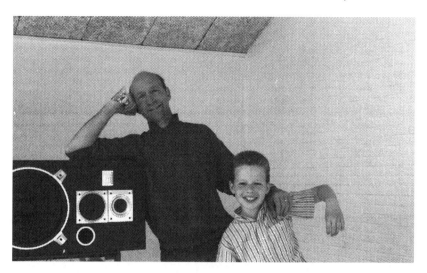

This is the only photo I have of Benjamin together with Mike. Taken in 1987, while we were redecorating the house in Bunschoten, the Netherlands.

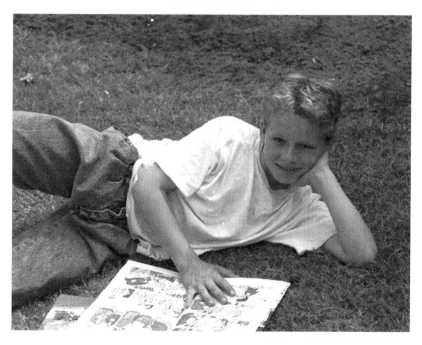

Benjamin reading one of his comic books outside in the yard. Benjamin loved comic books. Later when he was older he enjoyed reading non-fiction books and lots of them. Picture was taken in 1989.

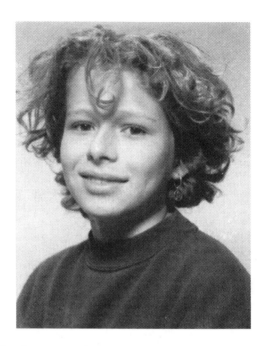

Another school picture. This one was taken during his second year in junior high.

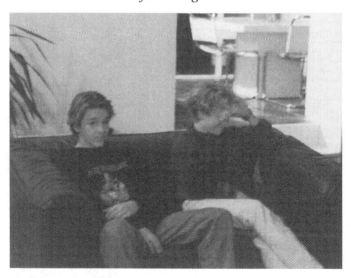

Together with his friend Klaas when we lived in Bunschoten, the Netherlands. Both are approx 13-14 years old here. Klaas was Benjamin's best friend. They first were buddies when they were only three years old. They remained friends until his death.

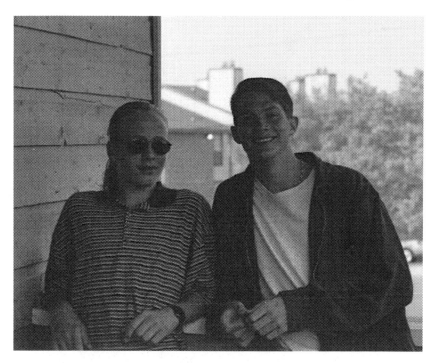

Austin Texas in 1994 with his stepbrother Kenneth. Together with Ken, a few years later, they first "stepped out into the world" by sharing an apartment together, learning to stand on their own feet.

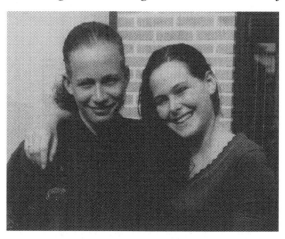

Another photo of Benjamin with his sister Zoë. Benjamin had long hair (tied back in a ponytail) during this period. His hair was just as curly as Zoë's. Photo was taken in 1995.

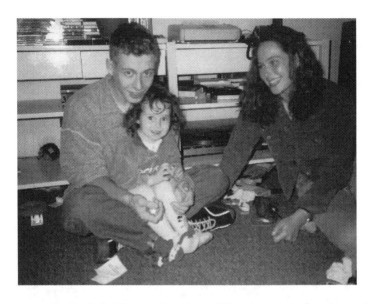

Benjamin, his little half-sister Sarah and Zoë in 1998. Sarah was born in 1996 when Benjamin was already living in the US.

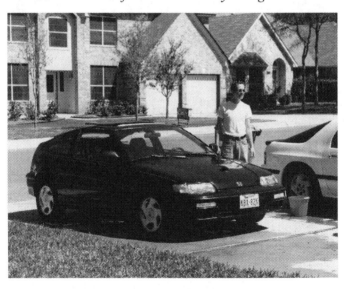

Benjamin with his first and only car he owned. Benjamin loved his little Honda Civic. This is the car he was driving when the police stopped him the night he had wanted to discuss with me that he thought he had cancer. The night they had thrown him in jail. Photo taken on the driveway of our house in Austin, Texas.

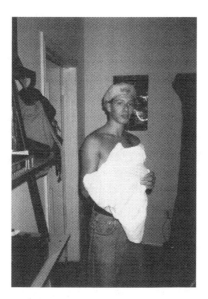

Austin Texas. Benjamin 19 years old. Strong and very handsome. No cancer yet.

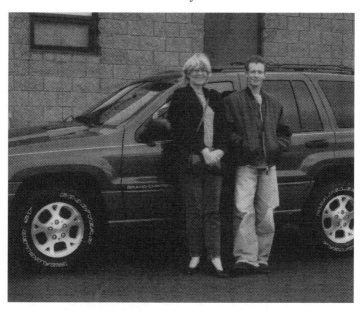

One of the very few photos of Benjamin and I together. This one was taken when we picked up our Jeep from the car dealer in New Jersey in August 1999. We had moved to New Jersey for his treatment. Benjamin had started Leatrile treatment.

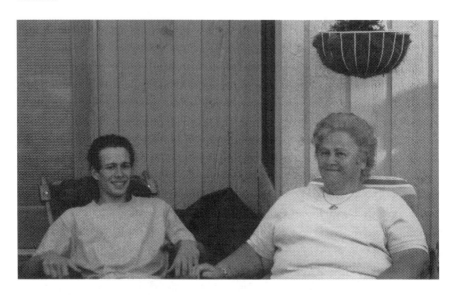

*New Jersey 1999. Benjamin together with his grandmother ("nana").
Still looking good and happy even though he had been diagnosed with
cancer earlier that year.*

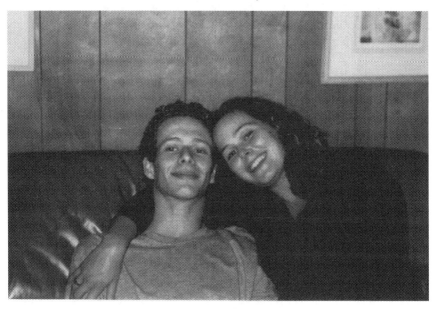

*Benjamin and Zoë. Taken when Zoë was visiting us and her nana in NJ
during the summer of 1999.*

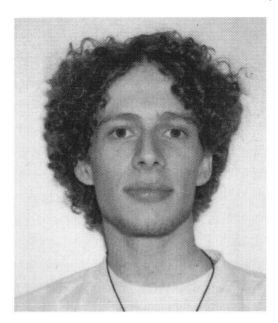

Benjamin just before he left to return to the Netherlands early 2000. He looked still pretty good, considering.

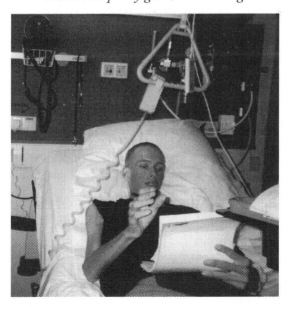

June 2000. In the VU Hospital in Amsterdam, the Netherlands. Altogether he stayed in the hospital a total of more than 2 months. It had been his worst nightmare.

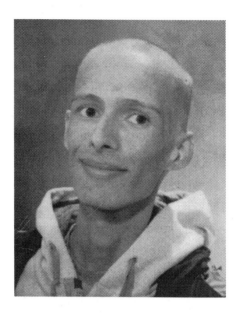

This is what chemotherapy did to Benjamin. After a couple of rounds there was barely anything left of him.

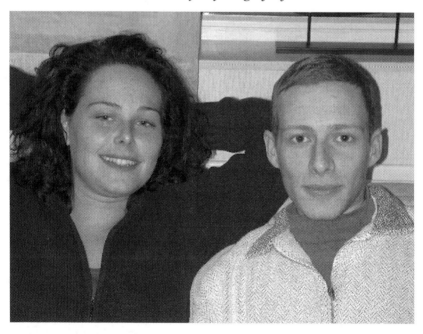

Regaining his strength and weight. Together with Zoë in the apartment I had rented in Amersfoort. Bit by bit Benjamin was getting better.

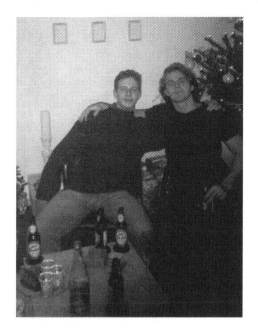

Celebrating Christmas with his friend Klaas in December 2000.

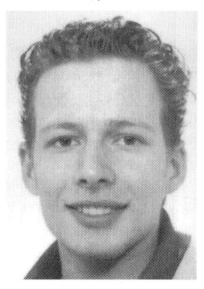

This is the picture Benjamin had had made for his Dutch driving license in April 2001. The picture we used for his "mourn card". He looked at his best here since his chemo. Taken during the period we thought he had beaten the disease.

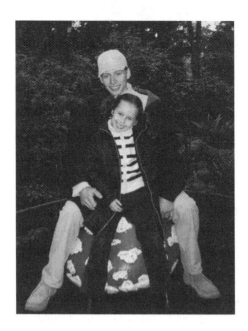

Autumn 2001. Together with his little sister Sarah during a day out in an amusement park. Benjamin died a month before Sarah turned 6 years old. The only regret he had… not being able to see Sarah grown up.

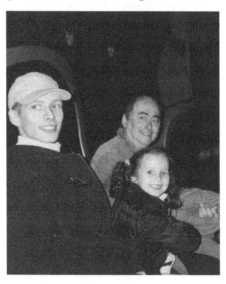

…and here together with his dad Wayne and his little Sister Sarah at the amusement park. These are the last pictures we have of Benjamin before he passed in February 2002.

CHAPTER 6

Recovery?

Here I am—the complete me
Hidden for so long behind mysteries and riddles
Afraid to live and now so close, afraid to die
Cancer? I never had cancer ...
I was at war ... at war with myself and with the world

Benjamin Hyman—July 2000

On Tuesday morning, May 16, 2000, I tried to call Zoë from my hotel before going to my consultancy job in Phoenix. Zoë was not home, but I spoke to Frido, her partner. As a gift from God, he gave me the good news. Benjamin had been admitted in to the VU Hospital in Amsterdam. Zoë was there with him. Benjamin was in the hospital getting medical care! This was the best news I had heard since many months ... A heavy load fell from my shoulders; *thank you, God, thank you*. Finally Benjamin had taken the steps we all wanted him to take: he would get conventional medical care. I was so relieved.

Soon after that fantastic phone call Zoë e-mailed me.

Dear Mama,

I am just back from the hospital, and as you already know from Frido, Benjamin has now been admitted. He is in the VU Hospital in Amsterdam. He has a phone and TV in his room, and he can call internationally. The oncologist that is treating him is called Dr. Klaas Hoekman. He claims to be the best in Europe—said to Dad to check it out on the Internet. We don't know where, but we'll find out. Perhaps on the VU's Web site, if they do have one? They have taken blood, and right now Benjamin is getting an IV with water and salt or something like that. Dr. Hoekman briefly explained what is going to happen. Tomorrow he will get CT scans of his entire body. Tonight they made an ultrasound of his leg, and they did diagnose thrombosis. I still need to check on the Internet to find out exactly what that means, and I still need to ask what they are going to do about it. He will get chemotherapy—the same protocol Benjamin saw on the BBC[34] a couple of days ago. Dr. Hoekman assured us that this type of cancer is easily and quickly cured. This particular type of chemo works extremely well for testicular cancer. Fortunately!

He will first get further medical checkups, and then they'll start with chemo. Most probably he'll get four to five cycles of chemo. One cycle consist of five days of therapy, then two to three weeks off, then again five days of therapy, again two to three weeks off, and so on, until he has been through this cycle four or five times. All together it will take approximately three months. But he will feel much better before the three months are over. And perhaps he can go home after a couple of weeks and be treated as an outpatient. I have seen a couple of people without hair; I don't know if they have been treated with chemo, but one young man Benjamin's age looked extremely well, as far as weight, etc., was concerned. I did not talk to him, though. I am going to get some things together for Benjamin. Also still have to inform everybody in our family that Benjamin has been admitted. Arjan[35] already knows.

Benjamin really would like you to come to the Netherlands as soon as you can. Perhaps you can just visit soon? At my work they are very understanding about the situation, so I don't have to worry about that.

---

34.   Benjamin apparently had watched a program of the BBC about testicular cancer and the chemotherapy protocol they used. This program had pushed him over to finally seek conventional treatment.

35.   Benjamin's cousin.

They wish us, but especially Benjamin, lots of strength. I am allowed to take as much time as I need. Did speak to Luuc today; he sends Benjamin tons of energy and is thinking of him. Benjamin did briefly talk to him. Luuc really wants to help as soon as Benjamin is stronger physically. Everybody is there for him and willing to help. He is going to make it. I am sure of that! I hope that I kept you up to date. Please let me know how we can reach you. Okay, if you still want to call tonight late that's fine. I will be going back at the hospital—visiting hour is over—but he has a room to himself and I can just come and go as I please. I have taken the rest of the week off. So tomorrow morning I will be back in the hospital again as well. I could stay overnight, but it is only ten minutes from where I live.

I love you, and I'll tell Benjamin that you love him tremendously. Hope that you will be here soon.
Love and kisses from me.

Zoë e-mailed me again in the middle of the night. She had just returned from the hospital. Everything was okay. Benjamin had received something to help him sleep. She hoped that he would finally have a good night's sleep. The night nurse would check on him four times. The next morning at 8:00 AM the doctor would be there and so would she. If I wanted to speak to her, she suggested that I call just before 7:00 AM her time. She had bought a small stuffed giraffe for Benjamin to keep him company through the night. Benjamin had gone to sleep with it. I was so grateful I had such a fantastic daughter who was so willing to do all this for Benjamin. No matter what, she would be there for her brother. He could count on her, always. Nothing was too much for her. It had been like that since they were children. Although Benjamin was only two years younger than she was, Benjamin was in her eyes her little brother. And as his big sister, Zoë was always there to protect him, to stand up for him. They were very close, not just as small children, but also now as young adults.

I felt guilty that I was not there, that I was not there sitting beside his hospital bed and supporting him while he had to battle and overcome this awful disease. I went out to buy get-well cards. I also bought a packet with some interesting small rocks from Arizona—Benjamin loved rocks. Anything to do with nature, he loved. I would mail the rocks and make sure I mailed a card daily. That's the least I could do while I was here and he in the hospital. I would try to call him on a daily basis, but with the time difference and being at a client's, I was not sure whether that was a possibility.

The same day Susan contacted me via e-mail. She was wondering how I and of course Benjamin were doing. It had been a while since we talked or since she had heard from me. She was not sure where on the map I was that week but would appreciate hearing how Benjamin was doing as soon as I had the opportunity. She and her family were all okay, busy with work.

By the end of the day I was able to give her an update on what was happening with Benjamin. I forwarded the message also to Paula and Benjamin's grandma. Susan replied quickly and thanked me for the information. Her prayers had been answered. She was going to try to call Benjamin in a couple of days. She wanted to know how long Benjamin would be in the hospital and wondered whether Wayne was in the picture. She knew Wayne and Benjamin had their differences but assured me that Wayne loved him very, very much. I also received another e-mail from Zoë:

Wednesday, May 17
Dear Mom,

It is just past 11:30 AM, and I just returned from the hospital. Here is a short summary: Spoke to Dr. Hoekman. He explained what is going to happen. Benjamin will get a CT scan this morning, from head to toe, which takes approximately one hour. Then he will be transferred to the oncology ward. Tomorrow he'll start his first chemotherapy cycle. This will last until Sunday, so four days in total. He will get the chemo Benjamin saw on BBC. They are going to make sure he will have as few side effects as possible. He may get some tingling in his toes and fingers. It is also possible that he will not be able to hear high tones and that he will feel sick and may even throw up. His kidneys and liver are good, according to the blood test. His tumor markers are extremely high … but that's not news. It is very positive that his kidneys are okay. They have to do the work soon to eliminate the toxic waste from his body. Together with the chemo he will receive lots of fluid, to make sure he will pee about six liters a day. I suggested he have his hair cut very short or shave it all together. I don't think he finds it important.

Dr. Hoekman started talking about preserving some of Benjamin's sperm, because the chances of becoming sterile after chemo were so high. Benjamin decided not to do this. Hoekman said he probably would have a hard time anyway, considering the physical state he is in. There is a 50 percent chance that he will be infertile after the chemotherapy treatments. Who knows, he may get lucky! I find it a shame on the one hand, but it is much more important that Benjamin gets better. After four days he will not get "anything" for sixteen days (so no chemo). Most probably he can go home after chemo … not just yet, after his first cycle, but perhaps afterward. They will keep an eye on his leg. If things go well he is allowed to go home and he will receive medication for the clotting. Apart from that they started talking about the expenses. Where could they send the bills? I told them about Blue Cross and gave them your address. They want a payment in advance … the costs per day are approximately fourteen hundred guilders. They want me to transfer (don't be shocked) 10,000 guilders by Friday. So I'll need your credit card details. I think I still have the number, but just in case. If he were not insured, the VU does have a "kitty," and they'll pay. Don't really know how it works, but basically it means that if they find someone needs medical care and he can't pay for it, they'll use the money in the "kitty." I hope you have the money and that you can claim it from your medical insurance. Otherwise we have to ask Oma[36] to lend us the money. The money is not important; we will figure something out (sounds a bit silly perhaps, but I hope you understand that what counts is that Benjamin gets better).

Klaas visited for a short while today. He will try to drop by as often as possible. He also felt that Benjamin is going to be okay. I have tried to comfort Benjamin and told him not to worry, everything is going to be okay. We will go on vacation in September. The doctor was here when I told Benjamin that, and Benjamin asked the doctor whether he would be able to. The doctor answered yes, and Benjamin asked him if he would be able to run across the beach, and again the doctor said yes. I think Benjamin does trust him. I called Gerda[37] this morning

---

36.   My mother, Benjamin's other grandmother.
37.   My sister. Benjamin's aunt.

and spoke to Kim[38]. The family has been informed (assume that Oma is aware now as well, but perhaps I should call her). Benjamin's address, by the way, is:

Postbus 7057

1007 MB Amsterdam.

Using the postbox number means the post gets delivered much faster. Add the floor number and his room number, though. The Web site is ww.azvu.nl. I have not had time yet to check it out. I am assuming that Dr. Hoekman is on that site as well. I am jumping from one subject to another, but that does not matter hopefully. Just hope you are informed again. I'll let everybody know what Benjamin's hospital address is. I am hoping he will receive tons of get-well cards to support him. Dad was visiting today as well. He is planning to come every day.

I'll make sure I am with him again tomorrow morning at 8:00. I have seen quite a few young people with bald heads. Dr. Hoekman said he would make sure that Benjamin gets a young man his age to share a hospital room. Hopefully he will share with someone who does have some positive things to say and perhaps does have the same type of cancer Benjamin has. I would think that that would be good for Benjamin. The doctor told me that all patients with testicular cancer are sent to the VU hospital. I saw a young man Benjamin's age getting into a car today. He was being picked up after his chemo, I think, for he was bald. He looked so much better than Benjamin. I now think that anyone who is bald has cancer. Perhaps that's is so in nine out of ten cases.

Bumped into a friend of Frido's downstairs in the hall. He told me his father had leukemia and had already had several chemo cycles behind him. He was doing extremely well and was healing. He also is on Floor Seven East. Well, I am stopping. Good night. If you want to call again tomorrow morning, just call at the same time.

I love you and perhaps I talk to you tomorrow morning.

P.S. Not really a summary, oh well …

I let her know that I would take care of the financials and that she did not need to worry. I was going to transfer money from my Dutch bank account, but because of the time difference and the fact I could

---

38.   Benjamin's cousin.

not fax from where I was I e-mailed both my sister and brother to ask if they would help me out until I was back in Austin again. I also asked Zoë if she could request the hospital to provide me with detailed invoices, as detailed as possible, because I knew the American insurance company would hassle me and that it was hard to claim money. Most of the time it took weeks, if not months. My sister responded the next day that she had wired the advance to the hospital. I thanked her via e-mail and promised I would give her a call that coming weekend when I was home again.

Because Benjamin was starting his chemotherapy treatment on Thursday I decided to call him and wish him luck. I got him on the phone when he had just started the cycle. Zoë was there with him. She had stayed the night in the hospital with him, trying to comfort and support him. She had not slept all night because Benjamin had kept her awake. He was doing okay but was very scared and worried. We did not talk too much, and he preferred that I call when he started feeling a bit better. I hoped that would be soon. His CT scan was okay; it showed no further "damage." The cancer seemed very much contained in the sexual organ region and the lower part of his body. I was thankful that the cancer had not spread throughout his body. I truly believed that Laetrile had helped him but that we messed up by not getting rid of the toxic waste. I was wondering what Dr. Schachter's thoughts would be on that. Perhaps I should contact him.

I flew from Phoenix back to Austin the next day, Friday, May 19. During the weekend Mike and I discussed the possibility of returning to Holland to live. Whether we were able to do so all depended on whether I could afford to leave my job with such short notice or whether I had to stay on another six months or so. Would my Blue Cross insurance pay for Benjamin's medical costs if I were to leave now? They were questions I did not have answers to yet. Benjamin, not yet covered by the national health system in the Netherlands, was still under my coverage. I knew that Wayne was working on it, but those things took time, especially in Holland. The fact that Benjamin was of British nationality did not help; it just made things more complicated. And I still had not received any positive response, or rather any response at all, from the Dutch Immigration and Naturalization Bureau.

Mike was ready to move. As a matter of fact, he saw it as a challenge. I think he was ready to leave his current job at Motorola, as he was beginning to get fed up with his role as desktop support. I, on the other hand, was not so sure about moving back to Holland to live. I was sure about going back, definitely. I needed to take care of Benjamin. But packing up everything and going to live there for good? I was wondering whether that was the right thing to do. Especially because, in the past, Mike had been back and forth a couple of times, because he had difficulties settling down in Holland. What would be different this time? Why did he think it would be no problem this time?

I called Benjamin, though not as often as I would have liked. When I did speak to him I could hear he was exhausted, which made talking to him difficult. On Monday, May 22, Benjamin finished his first round of chemo. He was now being "flushed." So far, so good. After three weeks of rest he would start his second round. He had not yet had any bad side effects. But that did not necessarily mean he would not experience any. The doctors were confident that he would make it, or so they told us. He was scheduled to get between four and six rounds of chemo, total. I prayed that the chemo would work for him and that he would get well again, so that we could put this nightmare behind us. I was happy that Zoë was so supportive and was staying with him in the hospital, day and night. He needed someone there to help him through this rough time. She was putting her own life on hold for him.

Benjamin wrote in his journal: "I am sure enough beginning to get confidence in the western medical science. I see my progress since I have been here in the hospital. Although I dare not yet to become too enthusiastic … I feel grateful for so many ordinary things and less ordinary things. For the people around me." A few days later he wrote: "Today was a day with both ups and downs. Like this morning: all by myself I got from bed to chair to table. And yet one moment later I realized I was not able to get up out of the chair. Then the loss of my hair … The bits of hope disappeared again. Zoë always makes me feel better. The connection, the bond that we share, will never, ever be broken."

I thought of Benjamin every minute of the day, feeling guilty I was not there for him. I spoke to Susan about feeling guilty. She thought about that statement and, because she and I are both Tauruses, she came to the conclusion that we live our lives in a perpetual state of guilt. She advised me to try *not* to. Every choice, every decision had led me to this very point in my life, and I was in a good place. It was just so tragic that cancer had fallen into my family, on my son. But he was an adult, he had free will, and all of his choices were quite simply those that he had chosen to make. All I could do now was to pray for his well-being and his quick recovery.

I thought of going over for a weekend soon, as I was working from home again that and the following week. After that I had to go to Connecticut for two weeks, beginning Monday, June 5. I was scheduled to fly out of Austin via Atlanta to New York JFK. So perhaps I could visit Benjamin the weekend before. I could leave Austin on Friday, June 2, and arrive in Amsterdam early Saturday morning. I decided to go for it. I arranged my flights to and from New York for my business trip and added an extra leg from New York to Amsterdam to New York. I booked a rental car at JFK for Monday, June 5, after I came back from Amsterdam so I could drive to my client in Connecticut. It was going to be a hectic weekend—lots of flying, little rest—but I could do it. I needed to go and see my son. I told Benjamin I was visiting soon, and he really looked forward to my visit. I talked to him on the phone again a couple of times, but he still sounded very weak.

Zoë picked me up at Schiphol Airport Saturday morning around 8:00 AM. I would stay with her in Diemen the next couple of days. She had an extra bedroom upstairs in the attic. It was a big room with a double bed—plenty of room for me. We went straight from the airport to the hospital. On the way she told me how much Benjamin was looking forward to seeing me. Although I had just visited him at the end of April in the clinic in Denmark, it felt like it had been months. I was pretty excited to see him again as well. I had really missed him. Not one day had gone by without me thinking of him. He was always on my mind.

I asked Zoë how he was doing, how he was taking his therapy. Zoë told me that he was okay, but he was very thin. She had spent the last three weeks, more or less full time, with him in the hospital. She spent the nights in his room, just to make sure he was okay and had someone near.

When we arrived at the hospital, we had to take the elevator to the seventh floor. Although it was early in the morning, quite a few people were already about. I greeted them, said hello, nodded. But strangely, nobody said anything. What kind of country was this? People did not bother to greet each other or say hi? In the elevator they just stared, either at the floor or up at the ceiling. I had forgotten what it was like to be back in the Netherlands again. People here had forgotten how to be kind and polite to each other. How different from Texas, where everybody said hello or started a conversation with you about anything, regardless of whether you knew each other. In Texas it did not matter whether you were a janitor or a vice president; people were just friendly and polite to anyone.

We got out of the elevator and walked into Benjamin's room. There he was, in bed, hooked up to all sorts of tubes. Monitors surrounded him; an IV was stuck in his hand. My dear, beautiful son, so sick … We cried and hugged, very happy to see each other. How thin and frail he looked … His hair was almost gone, his arms nothing but sticks covered with some skin. He almost looked as bad as the victims in concentration camps during the Second World War. But he was alive, and the chemotherapy was beginning to show results. His tumor markers had already gone down dramatically, and his pain was gone. He was no longer on painkillers. Benjamin was happy about that, as he had wanted to get off the painkillers for a very long time. He could not walk, though.

His legs had swollen up enormously, and Benjamin was very worried about his legs, I think more than about his cancer. To get the swelling down, his legs were all wrapped up in stretchy bandages. The medical staff and nurses were great, very helpful and available immediately whenever Benjamin pressed the bell. I salute them for their work. I would have never been able to do what they did, being there for patients day in and day out for twenty-four hours a day. I met his oncologist, Dr. Hoekman, and his assistants. He suggested that I spent the night there with Benjamin, as he felt a family member should really be by his side all the time. Zoë had been there for most of the time. Now it was my turn, and I was happy to give her a break. The room had a foldable guest bed.

I helped Benjamin whenever my help was needed and did what I could. He was eating well and, amazingly, was eating food that in the past he would never touch. What had made him change his eating habits? Later on I found out that the chemo had somewhat changed his taste. I was pleased he was eating well. He needed to eat well to put on weight and get his strength back. Besides ordinary meals three times a day, Benjamin also ate small packages of astronaut food, loaded with vitamins and minerals.

I was shocked by his physical appearance. His testicle tumor was very large and the skin was open, I assume from so much pressure from the tumor. He also had very large stretch marks on his stomach and legs, just like in pregnant women. The marks looked like a lion or bear had tried to scratch him. The stretch marks on his body were a result of the chemotherapy and the fluid IVs; his body had been badly bloated and the skin had stretched. During the night Benjamin woke up several times; the open wound bothered him and caused discomfort. The wound needed dressing quite a few times. Sometimes I would do it, other times a nurse, depending who was on call. Benjamin liked some more than others, and there were a few he did not really get on with.

The next day my mother and sister visited Benjamin. After they spent some time with him, I stepped out of the room with them, to say good-bye. All three of us stood crying outside of his hospital room. They had not known what to expect, and they were shocked at what they saw. It was heartbreaking. There is nothing worse for a mother or a grandmother than seeing a child or grandchild suffer. We wanted to make him better, take his heartache and worries away. We prayed that he would survive, that he would make it and get well.

I was supposed to return to the States on Monday, June 5, but fortunately I received a call from my manager at IMG that the project in Connecticut had been postponed a couple of weeks, and there was no hurry for me to get back. How lucky I was! That meant I could change my flight to a later date and stay with Benjamin for another week or so. I was pleased, and so was Benjamin.

Benjamin had been a great fan of a Dutch group called "Doe Maar."[39] He had become an admirer when he was only eight or nine years old. They had stopped performing years ago, but during 2000 they got back together for a number of concerts and had been performing in various places all over Holland. The 2000 tour was going to be their last tour, and the concerts were more or less their final performances. Zoë knew all the members of the band and had already been to a couple of the concerts. Their very last concert was in Rotterdam on Wednesday, June 7, which would be followed by a big party for invited guests only. Zoë thought it would be nice for Benjamin if he could attend that concert. If he could, the group would invite him to their party afterward as a guest of honor. But Benjamin was in no condition to sit or to walk. However, the hospital staff, together with Zoë, was willing to make it happen for Benjamin. They allowed him to go to the concert by arranging an ambulance for him.

And he did go. He attended the concert in an ambulance bed. His bed was placed right up front. A nurse went along and saw to it that he was safe and well. It was amazing what they did to arrange all this. Benjamin was very excited. Looking back, I realize that the hospital staff went out of their way to do this for him because they never thought he was going to make it; they did not believe he would get out of the hospital alive. The concert was a success. Benjamin enjoyed it tremendously; he had had his picture taken with the members of the band standing all around his hospital bed. They even captured him on video during the party. He met all the band members personally, and he got their CD autographed by them. During the party, he also received an invitation from the AJAX[40] director himself to attend a football game in August as the guest of honor.

The few times I did not stay overnight at the hospital, I stayed at Zoë's. That gave me a chance to catch up on my e-mails and to communicate with my relatives and friends in the United States. It also allowed me to check back and forth with my employer. Again I was told that I did not need to rush back because the project had been postponed again. In the end, the project was cancelled altogether. I changed my

---

39.   Roughly translated, Doe Maar means "But Do."
40.   AJAX is one of the greatest soccer teams in Holland

flight once more. I was glad, because it was obvious that I could not go back to the States while Benjamin was in this condition. I decided that I would stay in Holland, and I started looking for a permanent place to stay. I had discussed this with Mike, and Mike felt it would be better if we sold up in Austin and he, too, would move to Holland. I consulted several realtors in the Gooi- en Eemland area, where Benjamin was born and grew up.

It was not easy to find something because rentals went quickly, due to a very tight housing market in Holland. For a lot of people, buying a house had become unaffordable, and therefore rentals were hard to come by. But again I was lucky. In Amersfoort, new apartments were finished and had just come up for rent. One was left. The apartment had two bedrooms, a very large living/dining room, a big bathroom, and a workable kitchen. There were several elevators, so no need to worry about Benjamin climbing stairs. It was a very suitable location, in the center of Amersfoort above a new shopping plaza. Everything was within walking distance. Just below the apartments were the bank, a small supermarket, and the post-office, plus restaurants and major department stores. It could not have been more convenient. I grabbed the opportunity and signed a lease agreement. I could move in as of July 1.

Benjamin was scheduled to start his second round of chemotherapy on Friday, June 9. Then for a reason not known to me, Benjamin decided he wanted to leave the hospital. Wayne was visiting at the time. We tried to convince him that he needed to stay, that he was not in any condition to get up and walk. He had not been out of bed unassisted. He had only managed to walk a few steps with the help of somebody or with the help of a medical walker. But that did not stop him. He took out his IV, got up out of bed, and walked out of his room. We were stunned, and before we realized what was going on and what he was doing, Benjamin had walked down the hall toward the elevator. We tried to stop him, but he was stronger than we thought. As he approached the stairs, he fell to the floor. We helped him up and pleaded with him. He was in no condition to leave the hospital; we begged him to go back into this room. I told him I would return to the States if he was going to be like this, as I could not take it anymore, that I would not come back until he was well again.

He had really done it this time. Perhaps he was acting like this because he was afraid I would leave and he did not want me to go home. We tried to convince him that he needed to stick to the plan if he wanted to get better, but Benjamin was strangely unresponsive. Surely he realized, after all he went through the previous year and the state he was in now, that it was a matter of life and death. If he did not follow through this time he would surely die. Why was he doing this? I knew he hated the hospital, but he himself wanted to be admitted, and he himself had realized this was his last chance to survive. Was he playing games with us all, his only power now the power to torment? Or didn't he want to get better?

We did persuade him to stay, which was not difficult given his weakened state, but it was more than obvious that a family member needed to stay with him night and day. We continued to do so. Most of the time it was me. Sometimes his father would stay overnight. Benjamin began his second round of chemo but not without further struggle. At the beginning of his second round of chemo he decided he did not want further therapy, and he chose to cut the IV tube with a pair of scissors. The chemo spilled on the hospital room floor. This was bad: chemo is a very toxic and dangerous chemical. Cancer patients should not be in contact with it. Which makes you wonder why medical professionals dare injecting it into sick people's veins …

Not until recently, almost eight years later, when I read a medical report did I find out that the medical staff was giving Benjamin haldol[41] and dexamethason[42], both of which Benjamin did not need and were administered without my knowledge or any other family members' knowledge. No wonder he behaved the way he did. After the IV tube cutting incident, the doctors took him off dexamethasone. A medical social worker intervened and came to see him on a regular basis. It still

41.   Haldol (haloperidol) is indicated for use in the treatment of schizophrenia. Haldol is used to reduce the symptoms of mental disorders such as schizophrenia.
42.   Dexamethasone is used to treat many inflammatory and autoimmune conditions, e.g., rheumatoid arthritis. It is also given to cancer patients undergoing chemotherapy, to counteract certain side-effects of their antitumor treatment. Side effects a.o. psychiatric disturbances, including personality changes, irritability, euphoria, mania.

makes me sick to think what kinds of drugs have been administered without patient knowledge. Benjamin continued after this disaster and finished his second round of chemotherapy.

Benjamin wanted so badly to get out of the hospital that I discussed with the hospital staff whether he could go home after the second round of chemo and come back in when his third round was due, just like other cancer patients did. But Benjamin was not physically ready to be out of the hospital. Some members of the staff were totally against it; others were willing to let him go. He had been in the hospital now for over a month. It might do him good to leave for a couple of days. So as a trial, to see how things went and whether we could cope, we all agreed that Benjamin would go home for the weekend. Home this time meant staying at Zoë's, as she lived only ten minutes from the hospital. We agreed that if it did not work out, or if we needed medical assistance, I would call the hospital and we would return immediately. If things did work out, Benjamin would be discharged the next week until his third round of chemotherapy.

Benjamin and I stayed in Zoë's spare room, which was located on the third floor of her house, which was not really convenient, because it meant we had to climb two sets of stairs. Especially for Benjamin, that was very difficult. It meant I had to help him with every single step he took, a very heavy job. But I did not mind. I was only too glad to help him whenever I could. I was just glad that he was out of the hospital for a few days. We made the most of it; I tried to give him a good time. I drove him to see my mother, who was eighty-seven years old and still lived by herself in a bungalow. Benjamin asked if he could stay with her, because her house was just one story and everything was so convenient. She had a high toilet in her bathroom, with handles to hold onto. Her bedroom had tools that helped her get in and out of bed. The bed could be adjusted up and down automatically. It would have been perfect for Benjamin. But of course my mother was too old to be able to take care of Benjamin, even if only for the weekend. We just had to make do with Zoë's room in the attic for now. Of course we managed, and soon we would be in our own apartment in Amersfoort.

Mike was busy in the States. He had put up the house for sale. He was trying to sell all our belongings, as we did not think it was worth the cost to have everything shipped. Besides, we were moving from a large four-bedroom detached house into a small apartment. There was no room for our bulky furniture. It must have been tough on him; he had to take care of everything by himself. We tried to talk on the phone as often as possible, but that was not always easy.

There was so much to arrange, not just for him, but for me also. On top of that I needed to be in the hospital most of the time. Regardless, I also needed to get the apartment ready before July 1. In Holland, all leased apartments come totally bare: concrete floors, no lamps, no kitchen appliances, nothing. Before you can move in, you have to have flooring laid; you need a fridge, washer, dryer, etc. You need window treatments, lamps, plus of course furniture. I ordered laminate flooring for the entire apartment, bought a washer, dryer, stove, fridge, and dishwasher. A friend helped to put all the light fittings in, and my brother, who dealt in bankrupt stock, moved in some furniture, including a desk and office chair, dining table and chairs, and two leather lounge chairs. Without everybody's help it would not have been possible to do. I was happy that I had a desk and chair. At least I could now work from home remotely, until my company wanted me back on a project somewhere. I did not know how I was going to manage once they did call me, but that was to worry about later. Right now I needed to take care of Benjamin and make sure he had a good place to come home to, once they discharged him.

The hospital temporarily discharged him on June 20, but he needed to be back in from June 29 until July 4. Until the apartment became available Benjamin stayed with his father. A hospital bed had been placed in Wayne's living room, as it was too hard for Benjamin to climb two flights of stairs to his bedroom. A nurse came by a few times a week to help him with his bandages and to keep an eye on his thrombosis. In the meantime, we were moving Benjamin's personal stuff, including his bed and the sauna, into my apartment. I contacted my old e-mail friends in Canada, Australia, and England, as I thought I might be a good idea for Benjamin to daily take ozone steam saunas to help him with his health. All three of them agreed and instructed me about the temperature, the length of the daily treatment, and which supplements he should take.

Mike decided to just e-mail me from then on, because I was hard to get on the phone. He e-mailed me that the house had sold within a week. The contract was going to be signed on July 14, and the closing date was set for August 14. That meant I needed to be in the States then. He had called three different moving companies and had received estimates. He reported to me daily, letting me know what had been sold and what was probably going to be left over to be shipped. Sometimes I wondered whether I was doing the right thing. I knew that I needed to be in Holland for Benjamin, but I was not sure that selling everything in the States was the answer. I guessed time would tell.

Our relatives in the States were anxious to hear from us. They wanted to know how Benjamin was doing. Now that I was living in Holland I had not been e-mailing them as frequently as when I lived in the United States. They found not knowing what was going on very disturbing.

The third round of chemotherapy was concluded without problems, thanks to the fact that Benjamin no longer received dexamethasone. After he finished his third round, Benjamin moved in with me to the apartment in Amersfoort. He had looked forward to it. He had asked me to stay in Holland when I returned last month. He told me he needed someone to take care of him. He did not really want to go back and live with his father. Talking care of him was almost a full-time job. Benjamin needed assistance with everything. He was not able to get out of bed by himself, nor was he able to go to the bathroom by himself. He was still very, very tired every day and therefore not capable of doing much but rest. He got exhausted pretty quick and often told me that now he understood what it must be like to be an old man. He could walk maybe a hundred yards before he needed to rest and then continue. But he was doing better every day, bit by bit.

In mid-July I received an e-mail from Benjamin's American friend Kathleen. Kathleen was one of the few friends in the United States who knew Benjamin had cancer. He had not told all of his friends, and some of them did not understand why Benjamin had acted toward them the way he did or why he had left the United States all of a sudden. Kathleen, however, had known from the beginning, and she had kept in touch with him throughout the entire ordeal. She was letting me know she was planning to visit in a couple of months, but she did not want Benjamin to know yet, as she did not know exactly when she would be able to come over.

Around that same time I finally received word from the Ministry of Immigration and Naturalization, who informed me that Benjamin was not entitled to Dutch nationality. He needed to reside in the Netherlands again for five years before he could apply. That was totally ridiculous. Benjamin, my son, born in the Netherlands, born to a 100-percent Dutch mother, raised and educated here in the Netherlands, was not entitled to Dutch nationality? The Ministry was hopeless; they gave me no answers to all my questions. They just passed me on to other ministries and local governments. Typical!

Benjamin started his fourth and last round of chemo on July 21. He went back in the hospital for six days. Again this round was completed without too many problems, although before he went back Benjamin tried to convince me that he really did not need this fourth round. I don't think he felt he was really cured, but I do think he hated the hospital so much that he tried to convince himself he was already cured and that there was no need to go back.

We saw the oncologist. He was planning for Benjamin to have the operation to remove the testicular tumor around the end of August or beginning of September. The other tumors would not be removed, due to the risks associated with surgery. Regardless of what Dr. Andersen had told us, the chemotherapy had not shrunk Benjamin's tumors at all. None of them had been reduced in size.

After I took Benjamin to the hospital, my manager from the United States called, telling me that I was expected to be in Canada the next week. I had already been working remotely on this Canadian project, but now I needed to be present. So there I was, wondering what to do. I really did not have a choice; I needed to go and work until Benjamin had his surgery and the largest expenses would be behind us. I just did not know how Benjamin would react. I called Zoë, and she said she would look after him until I was back. She would move into our basically empty apartment. I also talked to Mike; I needed to be in Austin for the closing on our house on August 14. It was not a good time for me to travel, but then again I needed to stay employed so that

I was covered for health insurance. Benjamin was still not covered by the Dutch national health insurance; now that I had received word that he would not get Dutch nationality, I did not know how long it would take before he was covered.

I hated the thought that I needed to get back to the consulting business for the next six to eight weeks. It was time I started thinking about doing something else. I was always thinking of how I could start working for myself. In the States I had had several ideas about different opportunities. Perhaps the time had come to look into the possibility of materializing these ideas.

Benjamin finished his fourth round of chemo and was discharged from the hospital for good on July 26. He only needed to return two more times, as an outpatient, for an injection treatment called Bleo chemo. No more admittance was necessary for the time being, not until surgery in September. He needed to get back his strength and put on some weight. The chemotherapy did kill the cancer cells and reduced the tumor markers all the way down to where they should be. Benjamin was okay, but he looked worse than before. It seemed he went two steps back. This fourth round had really knocked him out and taken away his last bit of strength. He had no condition whatsoever, and he was pretty down. He could barely walk a block, and he weighed barely 100 pounds (45 kilos). It was absolutely necessary that he next began to put on weight and regain his strength. I needed to be there for him and make sure that he got into a scheduled routine of eating properly at least three times a day and that he got enough rest. Thank God he did not need further chemo.

He was pleased to be back with me in the apartment, pleased that I was taking care of him and not his father. He also liked the location where we were. It was convenient for him. He could take an elevator down, and all the stores were around him. This was great, because he could not walk very far and was out of breath in no time. Then I received word from my manager that I did not need to go to Toronto yet, but that I could continue to work remotely. I had been so lucky these past few months. Every time, things had worked out in my favor. At least I could spend all my day time with Benjamin. I could make sure that he ate well and got proper care. In the evenings and at night I worked on the Canadian project, sometimes until 3:00 AM. I was beginning to get exhausted, to the point that I took my frustrations out on Benjamin at times. I yelled at him when he was not communicating with me, when I did not know his needs. I shouted and cursed, and poor Benjamin just let me. I now feel terrible and very guilty about it.

I flew out to Austin on August 2 to take care of all sorts of details, sign over the house, and help Mike with the last bits and pieces. The couple of weeks in the States were hectic—so much to do in so little time. We needed to go through all our personal belongings, clothes, papers, books, etc., and decide what we would ship, what we would leave behind and give away. We decided to donate nearly two dozen cartons full of books to the local library.

On August 4, just two days after my arrival, I received a disturbing phone call from Benjamin. He had been to the hospital with his father for his last Bleo[43]. His oncologist, Dr. Hoekman, was not treating him, as he was on vacation. Another oncologist, Dr. Dercksen, was attending to Benjamin, and he told Benjamin that he was expected back into the hospital Friday, August 11, for his fifth round of chemo. He said Benjamin needed another two rounds. Dr. Hoekman, Benjamin, and myself had agreed a week or so earlier that Benjamin did not need another round of chemo. Instead Benjamin needed to get his strength back and gain weight for his upcoming surgery in September.

Benjamin was not happy about Dr. Dercksen's assessment and expressed his concern to me. I was not at all happy about this either and was deeply concerned, just like Benjamin, especially because the fourth round really harmed Benjamin, much more than the other three. Benjamin and I both felt that he would not be able to cope with two more rounds. It would be the chemo that killed him, not the cancer, if he were to receive two more rounds of poison. Anybody could see Benjamin would not last through it. I was also worried because I read up about the chemotherapy protocol used for testicular cancer. Standard protocol was either three or four cycles of BEP[44]. Poor risk patients typically received four cycles. Nothing was said about five or six cycles.

---

43. BLEO = Bleomycin, used as an anti-cancer agent
44. BEP = Bleomycin, Etoposid, and Cisplatin

I told Benjamin that I did not agree with Dr. Dercksen and that I would call him and talk to him. I also would try to contact Dr. Hoekman. I managed to get hold of Dr. Dercksen on the following Monday and talked to him on the phone. I explained my concern, and I listened to his advice and told him that I would discuss the different options with Benjamin and then let Dr. Dercksen know what we would do. He mentioned that he wanted to give Benjamin Carboplatin, which worried me because I read that you should never use Carboplatin to treat testicular cancer, except during a stem cell transplant. To make absolutely sure, I contacted an oncologist in the United States who Wayne had been communicating with and asked him for advice. In the meantime I also e-mailed Dr. Hoekman, hoping that although he was on vacation, he would read his e-mails. I expressed my concern to Dr. Hoekman and wanted to know why different approaches were being suggested; why was Dr. Dercksen insisting that Benjamin go for two more cycles? Anybody could see that the last round of chemotherapy had almost killed Benjamin. Everybody agreed that he looked much worse than before.

The American oncologist got in touch and assured me that nobody gives more chemo than the patient needs, but that sometimes the doctors don't always have a clear picture of how weak the patient actually is. That was definitely the case with Dr. Dercksen! Anybody who had not seen Benjamin for a while—and you did not need to be a doctor—could tell that exposing him to more chemo would kill him. But the oncologist did not really advise what to do, whether to go for the extra rounds or not. Benjamin and I went with our gut feelings and decided against more chemo. I was convinced we made the right decision.

I let some friends know that I was back in Austin and met with them. It was good to be back and able to visit with friends. But time flew by, and on August 14 we drove to Houston to stay overnight with my Dutch friend Toni. We dropped my car off there. We were going to leave it at her place until October, when we would return to the United States once again to celebrate Mike's grandmother's ninety-fifth birthday. On August 15, Mike and I flew back to Holland from Houston. Mike had not seen Benjamin since he left Austin in the beginning of March 2000. He did not say it, but I could see by his face and expressions that he was shocked when he saw Benjamin again. It was obvious he did not know what to expect, but he had not expected Benjamin to look so thin.

To me, Benjamin looked much better. Since he finished his last round of chemo he had already gained ten pounds, gaining that much in less than four weeks. Not bad. I hoped he would continue to do well and that he would have his strength back soon and be well enough for the operation. On the other hand, I was still worried about the tumor in his neck and the one in his abdomen. The one in his neck, which was visible, had definitely not become smaller; if anything it had become larger. Benjamin had been to the hospital for another CT scan, but we had not yet received the results. I hoped the scan would show that the tumor in his abdomen had been reduced. This tumor was beginning to bother him and now that Benjamin was putting on some weight, it felt uncomfortable. In the States, two ultrasounds had shown that this tumor was a soft tissue mass, but because this tumor was never biopsied, we never found out whether it was malignant or benign. The tumor in his testicle, which was the size of a large grapefruit, was becoming a nuisance.

Back in the apartment I tried to get back into a routine and get things organized again. It was harder with the three of us. Before I had just Benjamin to consider, but now there was Mike as well. I felt it as an additional burden. It was like having another child in the house. Mike did not speak any Dutch, so he also needed my help with certain things. He did not drive over here, as he did not hold a Dutch driving license, meaning that he depended on me for a lot of things. I was still "working" for IMG remotely once in a while, when there was remote work to be done. Because I told them I could no longer travel, my contract with them was going to end mid-September. After that, I would have no income. I approached Susan about whether she would be interested in starting a business with me. She and I worked on the business idea I had, or rather Susan worked on it. She did a lot of investigating and looked into a partnership that would be agreeable to both of us. I tried to make a commitment and work at the plan, but I realized that Benjamin still consumed most of my time and that the time was not right for me to dive into a business venture. Benjamin was my first and highest priority. Doing both, taking care of Benjamin and working on a business endeavor at the same time, did not work for me.

By the end of August we received word from the shipping company that our shipment was expected to sail on September 4 and would arrive in Rotterdam on September 24. I still had mixed feelings about living here in Holland again, especially together with Mike. In the past Mike had not liked it here, and that was exactly the reason he had moved to the States. I worried—why would it be different this time? But I needed to stay focused; my major purpose was helping Benjamin to get well again.

From the time Benjamin was discharged from the hospital, I had been trying to get reimbursed from Blue Cross for the submitted claims. I had submitted my last claim over seven weeks ago, but no word from Blue Cross. I called to find out whether my claims had been processed, but every time I spoke to someone I got a different excuse. I was told that my claims were not in the computer, that they were either still at somebody's desk or that they might be lost. It was impossible to get hold of anyone who had authority in that company; supervisors or managers were never available. None of the people at Blue Cross I spoke to could or would give me any names or phone numbers of people within the organization who could actually do something or respond to my needs. I was getting fed up with their services and their lack of expediting claims. I searched the Blue Cross Web site to see if I could find some names of managers or directors and their e-mail address. I did not want to deal with the customer service reps any longer; they were unable to do anything. They were obviously told to tell customers all the various excuses. Whenever I asked to speak to a supervisor or manager, nobody was available. They were either gone for the day, or they were no longer with the company, or whatever excuse they came up with. By searching Blue Cross' Web site I finally found names of the company's top people in the newsroom section. I also found an e-mail address for one of the PR people and forwarded an e-mail, hoping something would start happening after that. In the e-mail I quoted a sentence from their Web site, whereby Blue Cross claimed they offered unparalleled expertise in responding to customer needs. I wanted to know how it was possible that although I had submitted claims, I did not receive any reimbursements.

Finally I began to get some response, and then the ball started rolling. Within just a couple of days of e-mailing the PR staff, I started receiving good service from a couple of people at Blue Cross, and they helped me by processing the claims. However, it would take a while before I received any reimbursements.

By September 2000, Benjamin seemed to be doing okay. He had gained fifteen pounds since the beginning of August. However, I did not really know what to think. He had an appointment with the urologist on Friday, September 8, and another appointment with his oncologist the following Tuesday. In the meantime we had received the results from the last CT scan, which said that Benjamin's prognosis was bad. Supposedly he had multiple tumors in his abdomen and also between his lungs. However, they could well be benign, because his tumor markers were way down. Some of them were totally back to normal. The tumor in his neck was biopsied again, and they took an ultrasound. I was there and saw on the monitor how the neck tumor looked on the screen. It looked like fluid-filled chambers, like a bunch of grapes that were cut open. We still were waiting for the results. Not knowing whether these tumors were malignant or benign plus the bad prognosis was getting to me—and not just me. I could see by his behavior and moods that it affected Benjamin. I could only imagine what it meant for him, because he never talked to me about how he felt, how all the prognoses and results impacted him. He never complained, and he never expressed his concerns. I wished he were more open with his feelings. I could not understand why he wasn't more active, especially now that he was gaining some of his strength back and could get around a bit better. Why didn't he go out for walks more; why didn't he exercise on the home trainer equipment to build up some muscle? I did not find out until later that although he was not as much in pain, he was uncomfortable all the time. Sitting or standing was awkward and very uncomfortable because of that big tumor in his abdomen, so he would lie down most of the time.

In mid-September our belongings from Austin arrived—not all that much, because we sold most of our furniture, yet we still managed to ship seventy-five boxes of bits and pieces. The most important things were our desktop computers and printers. I had had only my laptop from IMG. But because I was no longer employed, I needed to get that back to them somehow. We had ADSL installed, which was nice because I could log in without blocking the telephone line and pay a fixed fee instead of by the minute. Benjamin was scheduled to have his testicle removed the first week of October, but he was hesitant and wanted some more questions answered by the specialist before moving forward; specifically, he wanted to know how much surgical experience the specialist had and how the surgery would be performed. He had not felt comfortable with the specialist and wanted to know more about him before undergoing the operation. He really wanted to cancel the operation. I thought he should go ahead and have it done. I decided to contact those who had given me helpful advice in the past. I needed not only input from the specialist who was going to operate on Benjamin but also to hear what my international doctor friends had to say. I e-mailed them all to let them know how Benjamin was doing and that he had completed his four rounds of chemotherapy. I explained that his tumor markers had gone down to almost normal, his HCG was already below five, and the AFP was now nine, although his tumors had not decreased in size. I told them that Benjamin was not in favor of having his testicle removed; what did they suggest he do?

Besides the operation, the hospital wanted to give him another two rounds of chemotherapy after the operation to see if the extra rounds would shrink the tumors. Benjamin and I both believed that he should not have another two rounds of chemo. Why put all that poison in his body just to see if the tumors would shrink? If they hadn't shrunk yet, we felt another two rounds would not do it either.

I received answers from them all. Saul replied that he recommended removing nothing. He said all Benjamin's parts were right where they should be. The problem was the toxic buildup, which starved the cells of oxygen, forcing them to ferment their sugar in order to survive. "Removing body parts does nothing to remedy the cause," he wrote. Furthermore, he said that the doctors knew it was going to come back, because it always does if you don't clean out the toxins. "That's why they want to do more chemo now, to make a few more dollars before it hits again, and put your son in his grave. Don't be fooled. It is taking a breather and will be back in spades." Now was the time, he said, to do the maximum amount of saunas and funneling. "When it comes back," he wrote, "it will be twice as hard to get rid of."

Following Saul's advice, Benjamin used the ozone steam sauna daily. I truly believed that if we had paid more attention to Dr. Schachter's protocol and had we done more to get rid of the toxic waste when Benjamin was on Laetrile, he would have been cancer-free by then. The beginning of October came and went. Benjamin never went for the operation. He had decided not to have the surgery at this time. He felt he was still too weak to have an operation. Besides, Dr. Andersen from Denmark had suggested it was not necessary and that Benjamin should leave it alone if he could cope with it. At first I was totally against Benjamin canceling the operation. I spent one full day trying to convince him he needed to have it done. I talked to him until I was blue in the face. But Benjamin would not be Benjamin, and if he did not want to do something, he did not do it. From that moment on I decided that I was no longer going to try to change his mind. It was his choice.

Then I read in the medical report that the doctors were only going to remove the testicle for research purposes, nothing else. The medical report said: "For palliative reasons, we plan to remove the primary tumor (right testis). The continuation of chemotherapy will take place afterward, if the patient agrees." But Benjamin did not agree. He made up his mind he was not going to have any more chemo. I supported him in his decision.

I continued spending a lot of time trying to get reimbursed by Blue Cross. It had become almost a full-time job. I wrote e-mails back and forth and was involved with a handful of helpful people within the organization. Finally in the beginning of October I received word that they would process my claims at the out-of-network level, which meant they would only pay 80 percent. I did not agree with this, as it had been an emergency when Benjamin was admitted to the hospital here in Holland and therefore they should pay 100 percent. My policy covered 100 percent out-of-network emergency. Besides, medical treatment in Holland was much cheaper than in the United States. They should be pleased he was treated here—it saved them money. And they were only willing to pay 80 percent? I was disgusted, and I was just not going to accept it without a fight.

Because I no longer had a paying job, I needed to start thinking about what I was going to do for a living. I tried once more to work on the business plan Susan and I had discussed, but again I could not get myself going. The proposed business venture was to market a device that would save big retail companies a lot of money. Susan had already done a lot of groundwork in the United States. The next step was for me to prepare a proper project plan. However, my enthusiasm and energy levels came and went in spurts. One day they were up, the next day they were down, like a rollercoaster. I wanted to get both Mike and Benjamin involved and get them to work on this as well. But it was like having to pull everybody along. If I did not do anything, nobody did anything. It was costing me too much energy, pulling me down.

In the end, the business endeavor did not work out. Looking back, the time was not right; I had too much on my hands and on my mind. Once in a while I still worked remotely for IMG and was paid only for those hours that I worked. It did not add up to much, but every little bit helped. In the meantime IMG wanted me to come to Philadelphia in November for a meeting to discuss the future of IMG Americas.

Mike and I were planning to fly to the United States on October 11 to celebrate his grandmother's ninety-fifth birthday. We planned to stay in the United States for one week only. Zoë would look after Benjamin while we were gone. Apart from the birthday party and family reunion, I also needed to go back to the States to take care of some unfinished business. I needed to ship my Jeep Cherokee Laredo, which was still in Houston, to New Jersey. Susan's daughter Michelle was going to take it over. It was good to have a break away from my day-to-day routine at home. We had a wonderful week in Texas. We visited with family and friends. We went to see our old neighbors and did some shopping.

Before we knew it we were back in Holland again. The week had flown by. Even though it had been short, the getaway had done me good. When we got back home, Benjamin looked good. His hair had grown a bit more, and he had put on another two pounds. He had continued with his daily saunas, and one of the abdomen tumors which was palpable on the right side of his lower back was beginning to look like a large boil or pimple. It was getting red and was painful because of the pressure. The skin began to peel. Benjamin saw our family physician, who thought it was an abscess and needed to be cut open to let the stuff out. I contacted my Canadian holistic doctor to see what his thoughts were on this. Saul told me that the ozone sauna was doing its work. "It's working—don't stop. Leave the boil alone. It will pop when it is ready. Nature knows what to do," he said. He had witnessed this before: a tumor took the course of least resistance and emerged through the skin. He advised us to let it drain and to use some hydrogen peroxide to keep the area around it sterile. We followed Saul's advice to also cup the tumor outside the sauna. Benjamin took daily ozone steam saunas. I helped him by cupping the tumor outside the sauna every night. Then the tumor burst open—nature was doing what it needed to do, getting rid of the toxic waste and removing the tumor. Neither this tumor nor the others had decreased in size during the chemo treatments. Benjamin and I were hopeful the tumor would now disappear.

We felt positive. I was wondering about what his oncologist had said. According to him, the cancer would come back. They were not going to remove the tumors because there were too many; the prognosis was bad. However, I was convinced Benjamin was going to make it. I never doubted that he would not get through this. The oncologist did not know that Benjamin sat in the ozone sauna, nor did he know that Benjamin still continued with his alternative therapies. Recently Benjamin had started seeing a physiotherapist to help him with his posture. He was not walking straight, because he was trying to avoid the pressure and discomfort the tumor in his abdomen was causing. Now that the tumor had opened, the pressure was decreasing. The tumor started discharging some kind of fluid, a clear liquid. Later it became more solid and yellowish, like pus, then a couple of days later it started discharging a pink-brownish-colored crud, like flesh. The pain vanished, and it was obvious that the tumor was shrinking.

The tumor continued discharging big pieces of tumor flesh. I took pictures of what came out because I felt if I told anyone, no one would believe me. Tuesday, October 31, 2000, we went to the hospital to see Benjamin's oncologist and for some more blood tests. His oncologist was quite nice for a change. He took a look at Benjamin's wound and realized it was dead tumor tissue. He immediately called for a surgeon to have a look at it and to see what needed to be done about it. He said he had never seen a case like Benjamin's. The surgeon suggested that Benjamin have himself admitted to the hospital next day so that they could cut it out. She said the wound would never heal by itself, and it would only get bigger. I asked her if she had seen anything like this before, and she admitted she had not.

Benjamin would not be Benjamin … and of course he declined the invitation to have himself admitted. Benjamin and I were sure that as soon as all the dead tumor tissue had been discharged, the wound would heal itself. It already looked like most of it had come out. The tumor was no longer visible from the outside. Benjamin felt much better because the tumor was no longer in his way; the pressure was gone. The wound continued to discharge for several months. In the end it did heal itself and closed up again without any interference from the medical world.

The month of November was rather quiet. We all felt somewhat at ease, because nature, taking its course had eliminated the large tumor. We felt confident that we would see similar results with the other tumors. We felt Benjamin was on the road to recovery. He was still gaining weight—so far he had gained over twenty pounds. His hair was almost all back, and he looked better every day. I did not worry as much anymore. We started to have time to begin to enjoy life in Holland.

Benjamin also began to enjoy life, bit by bit. It was still hard for him to walk very far. He was out of breath quickly, but compared to when he first left the hospital, he was a 100 percent better. He was still seeing the physiotherapist weekly to help him with his posture and to help him get back his strength. He sat in the ozone steam sauna daily, and he went as an outpatient to the hospital for blood tests. We got his blood test results back during the first week of November, and all tumor markers were normal. That was very good news. Benjamin still had a long way to go, but I was sure he would make it. Hopefully by next year he would be well and strong enough to start some kind of work or project, or perhaps go back to school. He started going out once in a while during the weekends with Klaas and Zoë.

I was still not working and never made up my mind what I wanted to do. I felt as though I was at a crossroad, not knowing where I wanted to be, not knowing which way to go. I missed the enthusiasm and energy to go forward that I used to have. I felt after one and a half year of worry and concern about Benjamin and moving from one place to another, I had reached a stage where I was at a loss. *Maybe I should give myself some time to relax and let it be for now*, I thought. For now, we were living off our savings, and the thought of going back to work did not yet appeal to me. I finally had some time to do things that had been put on hold since I had returned to Holland, such as pursuing medical insurance for Benjamin, purchasing a car, and getting rid of the very old, small car my brother had given me.

By the beginning of December, after Benjamin's wound had been discharging dead tissue for more than six weeks, I contacted Saul again. The chunks of tissue from the tumor in his abdomen were not that big anymore, and the wound now looked like a dimple instead of a bump. I wanted to know what we could do about the other tumors: the one in his neck and the testicle tumor. I wanted to know if the testicle tumor would ever disappear and shrink in size. It was quite large, the size of a grapefruit, and so far nothing seemed to have changed its size. Benjamin cupped that tumor in the sauna daily.

Saul wanted to know whether the testicular tumor was fluid or whether it was solid. It was solid. He suggested that we place a Glad sandwich bag around the scrotum. Then we should insert the ozone tube into the bag, set the flow at a certain rate, and have Benjamin sit in the sauna for twenty-five to thirty minutes. That way we would be sure that the maximum ozone went to the right place. For the neck area, we needed to try to make an enclosure around the tumor area, perhaps using a sandwich bag of light plastic, and tape it so that the tumor was surrounded. Then we could insert the tubing to deliver the ozone.

I also let Saul know that Benjamin had developed an itch and some kind of rash—it looked like small blisters—just above his butt. I wanted to know if Saul recommended that we continued the daily saunas. Benjamin had been using the sauna now five days a week for quite a few months. According to Saul, the itch and rash were released toxins, and that was good. He suggested we continue the daily saunas. Looking back, we should have been much more aggressive with the saunas, especially with cupping the visible tumors.

December was another pretty quiet month. I stayed in touch via e-mail with my American friends and tried to contact my Dutch friends, those with whom I had socialized before I moved to the States in the early nineties.

In mid-December I received an e-mail from Dr. Schachter, asking for an update on Benjamin. In the past I had been pretty good about letting people know how Benjamin had been doing. Over the past year and a half I had been in contact with very many doctors all over the world. All of them had been wonderful and very helpful. Now that Benjamin was on the road to recovery, I'd fallen behind with staying in touch and sending updates on Benjamin. I was glad to hear from Dr. Schachter and e-mailed him back the latest news: Benjamin was feeling much better since his body had eliminated the tumor. He was now able to walk much straighter and able to sit up better. I told him that Benjamin looked good, that his hair was back, and that he was happy. As a matter of fact, I had not seen him so happy and cheerful for a very, very long time. I felt that perhaps Benjamin was beginning to realize that he might have a good chance of beating this awful disease.

Dr. Schachter wanted to know what Benjamin was doing apart from the ozone saunas. Was he taking any supplements, was he on a special diet, did he have any other detox procedures? What did his blood work look like aside from the cancer markers? Benjamin was taking supplements but not that many. He took a multivitamin, and he drank Essiac tea daily. He took MGN3 and astragalus. Benjamin was not on a special diet, but I cooked daily and tried to cook healthy and sensible food. Organic produce was not readily available like it was in the United States. I did not know what his blood work was like, apart from the tumor markers. Nobody had done extensive blood tests as Dr. Schachter had done, as far as I knew. Benjamin no longer used Laetrile.

During the holiday season, Benjamin's friend Kathleen from Texas came. It was her first visit to the Netherlands. We celebrated Christmas at home in our small apartment, together with Benjamin, Kathleen, Zoë, and Frido. We were thankful to be together and that Benjamin was getting well again and recovering from his awful disease. Kathleen and Benjamin had a nice time together. They visited with Benjamin's friends, went sightseeing, and walked in the nearby forest. They enjoyed the snow in the park. We hadn't had snow for years in Holland, and for Kathleen it was a nice surprise. I believe she had never seen real snow in her life. During New Year's Eve, Kathleen and Benjamin went out partying, together with Klaas and Mariska, Zoë and Frido. They stayed overnight at Zoë's in Diemen.

I was so pleased they had a good time and that Benjamin had begun to pick up his life again and to be a joyful, healthy young man once more; he no longer had to carry that heavy load on his shoulders. It was very noticeable that he was pretty happy, very cheerful. He did not seem to be worried so much anymore and was not so serious anymore either. The old year, 2000, with all its misery, pain, and heartaches, left with all the fireworks. Benjamin and myself were looking forward to a healthy and happy new year. Benjamin deserved to be happy; he deserved a better life.

Over the years it had become a family tradition to visit my parents on New Year's Day. We would visit from early in the afternoon until the evening. Everybody was there: my brothers and sisters, in-laws, our children. Even though my father had passed away early 1990s, we had kept the tradition. Because I had moved to the States, I had not been there over the past seven years or so to celebrate the New Year with them. The get-together usually started with watching the New Year's concert from Vienna, Austria. We would drink champagne and eat the traditional Dutch *oliebollen*, a kind of round donut with raisins, without the hole, to toast the New Year and wish each other good health and a Happy New Year. We also ate different kind of cheeses and crackers, as well sweets, such as chocolates. There would be coffee and later wine and beer. My mother would make the traditional Dutch potato salad, made of potatoes, diced ham, apple, cooked red beet, pickles and pickled onions, hard boiled eggs, mayonnaise, which was served around dinnertime on a bed of lettuce and nicely decorated. It is eaten with slices of French baguette. It was nice that Benjamin, Mike, and I were there with them—the family was complete for the first time in years. I had strong hopes for the future and for Benjamin.

After the holidays Mike and I tried to get back into a daily routine. There were just the three of us in the apartment. We started with cleaning the place and taking the Christmas tree down in January. The snow had gone. It had been raining for a couple of days, and the temperature started rising. No more frost, no more snow. We received cards and e-mails from friends to wish us a happy and healthy New

Year. The days began to lengthen again, a bit every day, until June 21, when summer would start. I filled my days with daily chores. And I spent a lot of time behind the computer, staying in touch with friends overseas. I communicated with my friend Moe, whose sister had been battling cancer as well. She had been at it for three years and would not give up either. The cancer had not changed her spirit or attitude one bit. She was still undergoing chemo. Moe said she wanted to come and visit me this year. Now that we were living in Holland, a lot of my American friends wanted to come over and visit; that was something to look forward to that year.

I also updated my resume, as I needed to start thinking about work again. I was living off my savings, and money was beginning to run out. It was clear I needed to get back to work within the next few months. Although I rather liked being a mother and housewife, I placed my resume online and started to get responses from different companies and some headhunters. They were interested in me as a consultant. Lots of companies were looking for people with my particular skills. I would have preferred that Mike find a job so I could stay home and look after Benjamin to make sure he ate well and put on weight. But that was not to be.

During January I received several e-mails from Kathleen. She wanted to ask my advice; she was trying to figure out what her options would be if she moved to the Netherlands. She had liked it over here and cared deeply about Benjamin. I think it was more than just caring. I think she was actually in love with Benjamin. Benjamin liked Kathleen as a friend but did not want a loving relationship with her. He liked her because he could talk to her and have intelligent conversations with her. I don't think Benjamin was in favor of her moving to Holland.

Kathleen, however, was seriously looking into the possibilities. She had even contacted the Consulate General of the Netherlands in Houston. However, she was told that she would not be allowed to come to live and work in the Netherlands unless she were a doctor or some other "high-need" professional. Kathleen was a teacher, but she realized that teaching here in the Netherlands was not an option unless she could get a teaching job at an international school. Currently, no such openings were available. I stressed that before she could make such a step of moving over here, she needed to be absolutely sure that this was what she wanted to do, because living in a foreign country can be tough. It usually takes at least a year before you feel settled and at home. I knew from experience. In the beginning I was not at all happy in the States. I constantly wondered whether I had made the right decision and often thought of going back to Holland. I had the same feeling when I first moved back to Holland again the year before. It took me a while to feel at home again here in my home country. But the more Kathleen thought about moving, the more she wanted to do it. She had discussed it in depth with her parents, and they were very supportive.

I also e-mailed Susan a lot. We had not given up on starting a business venture together. *Perhaps now that Benjamin was getting better and did not need my attention so much,* I thought, *I could start thinking about this again.* I searched the Web for business connections; I looked into related opportunities and also at health-related opportunities.

I was looking up articles on Laetrile when I came across a disturbing news article about the Food and Drug Administration's crackdown on Laetrile's resurgence. The FDA declared Laetrile illegal and announced that a U.S. district judge had issued a preliminary injunction halting sales by three Internet sites; it warned consumers to be aware. What nonsense was this? Are people total idiots? How can a natural product like an apricot seed be dangerous? I wondered where people's common sense was. The FDA was declaring Laetrile illegal, while it was okay to pump deadly toxins into people's bodies. Benjamin was living proof that Laetrile did work and that it had not harmed him in anyway[45]. As a matter of fact, when Benjamin was on Laetrile he looked better than when he was on chemo. The FDA did not want people to take products that had not been proven to be safe and effective? Was chemo safe and effective? The article disgusted me. Why didn't the conventional medical world work together more often with the alternative medical world? Both could learn from each other.

During the day, after I had taken care of Benjamin and done all my household chores, I searched the Internet a lot. I looked around for job and business opportunities for myself and for schools and/or jobs for

---

45.   Philip Binzel Jr., MD, "Laetrile and the Life-Saving Substance Called Cyanide," www.worldwithoutcancer.org.uk/laetrileandcyanide.html; Pelton, *Alternatives in Cancer Therapy*; G. Edward Griffin, *World without Cancer: The Story of Vitamin B17*, 2nd ed. (Westlake Village, CA: American Media, 1997).

Benjamin. Hopefully some time soon, Benjamin would be able to start working again, or perhaps continue with his studies. For now he spent a lot of time behind the computer as well. He was learning applications, such as Flash and Dreamweaver. I forwarded Benjamin a link about a college that offered a three-month course that helped you identify what it was you would like to do, so that you could select the proper studies. He considered going to that school. Benjamin no longer had an idea of what he wanted. It seemed his dream of studying Chinese medicine had disappeared.

In the meantime I was overwhelmed with telephone calls for SAP consultants. I was surprised to see that they were willing to pay a lot of money for a SAP consultant. I also tried to help Zoë during that period. She had found a small store she wanted to rent to start a business. She had always wanted her own clothes store. She had talked to the owner of the store and was very enthusiastic about it. We worked together on a business plan. Further negotiations were needed before she could close a deal. The store was in a perfect location near where she lived, close by a supermarket. That coming weekend Zoë was to offer a bid on the store. She mentioned borrowing money from both me and my mother to get her going; she did not think the bank would finance her, as she did not have any collateral. If the deal materialized, she was considering opening in March or April. She was excited about it. Perhaps Benjamin could help in the store part-time for the time being, until he figured out what he really wanted to do with the rest of his life. We needed to wait and see how things would progress.

Toward the end of January Benjamin's oncologist called to see how Benjamin was doing and ask whether the wound had closed up. Benjamin visited his oncologist on Tuesday, January 30, 2001, and had another blood test. The results would be ready a couple of days later.

February 2 was Benjamin's twenty-third birthday. Zoë arranged a surprise party for him and invited about thirty friends he had grown up and had gone to school with before he moved to the States. He had not seen a lot of these friends since he returned to Holland in May. Only a few of them had visited him while he was in the hospital. Besides Klaas and Mariska, only one other friend had visited him here in Amersfoort. That was when Benjamin had just been discharged from the hospital.

At that time he weighed no more than a hundred pounds, and his friend had been totally shocked when they met. Although he had not expressed his shock to Benjamin, I could see it in his eyes. Half a year later, Benjamin looked good. He now weighed over 150 pounds, more than when he had been in the States. Apart from a couple of scars on his forehead, caused by the chemotherapy, you would never know he had been such a sick young man, that he almost died eight months earlier.

During the day of his birthday, Zoë took Benjamin out; she planned to be back around 8:30 PM. We had invited the friends to arrive around 8:00 PM. Mike and I made sure we went out to get all the drinks, snacks, and other party stuff while Benjamin was out with Zoë so that he would not suspect something was going on. It worked out well. The party was a tremendous success. We had fun. Benjamin was totally surprised, and it was good to see so many of his old friends again. His father and little sister Sarah were also here. Sarah was a really cute and happy five-year-old child. She now began to realize that I was Benjamin's mother. In the beginning she did not know where to place me. She could not really understand the relationships. She had a different mother than her sister Zoë and her brother Benjamin. The last guests did not leave until three the next morning.

On February 2, we had expected a phone call from Benjamin's oncologist to let us know the blood test results. However, he never called. A bit worried, I called the hospital myself that afternoon, only to find out that Dr. Hoekman was not available that day. His replacement was absent when I called, and he could not return my call for some reason. I asked if perhaps he could send me an e-mail with the results, but apparently the replacement had objected to that because Benjamin was not his patient. I was advised to call back the next Monday and speak to Dr. Hoekman himself. I did not like the sound of that. What was so difficult about letting us have the results now?

That same day I also received word from a recruiter that I was expected to start as an SAP consultant at a company in Sassenheim the following Tuesday. Sassenheim is approximately eighty-five kilometers from Amersfoort, which under normal circumstances would mean roughly an hour drive. In January I had been talking to several recruiters and consultancy firms and in the end had accepted this consultancy job in Sassenheim; it sounded as if they were flexible and would let me work four days rather than five if necessary. And occasional remote work might be an option as well. It was going to be hard to get back into the routine of getting up early and going to work. I was not really ready for it, but I had no choice; my money was running out, and I needed a regular income.

On Monday, February 5, we received the blood test results. The results were not good, although the HCG tumor marker had remained normal. Benjamin's AFP[46] tumor marker had risen from nine to twenty. That was too high. It should have been less than ten, preferably less than five. I was shocked, even though for some reason I had anticipated this. I had a premonition the results were not going to be good, perhaps because the replacement oncologist last Friday had been unwilling to share the results. I was worried. Right away I contacted my international friends again to ask for advice. The oncologist was undoubtedly going to advise more chemo. They had wanted Benjamin to have more chemo right from the beginning, without wondering whether his body was capable of handling more poison. Dr. Hoekman suggested we wait until the next blood test at the beginning of March before making a decision whether to go for chemo or not. I needed to know what Dr. Schachter and Saul plus the others thought about this and what they advised us to do.

Dr. Schachter let me know that recently he had become interested in a new nutritional approach called controlled amino acid treatment (CAAT). He thought this might be appropriate for Benjamin if the disease began to get out of control. In the meantime Benjamin should get back on the apricot seeds daily: between five and ten seeds four times a day. He should also start taking Megazyme Forte or Wobenzym enzymes[47]. Saul advised us to continue with the ozone saunas five days

46.   AFP is a marker for hepatocellular and germ cell (nonseminoma) carcinoma, while HCG is a marker for human chorionic gonadotropin (HCG) for gestational trophoblastic tumors and some germ cell cancers. There are many different types of tumor markers, but for testicular cancer AFP and betaHCG are used to measure the cancer.

47.   Enzymes are proteins that regulate digestion, production of energy, immune system activity, hormones production, and other body secretions. They aid in the destruction of foreign substances and protect us from deadly bacterial infections. Megazyme Forte may help maintain and support cardiovascular and lymphatic health, as well help support the immune system. Wobenzym has been found to degrade

per week. He felt as long as Benjamin's body was discharging fluid, the tumors would not grow. There was obviously a lot of material to release. Looking back, I realize that the AFP went back up again soon after the tumor in his abdomen had started closing up. No other tumor had started discharging, but no other tumors had been cupped as aggressively as that one. Both Benjamin and I were rather depressed after we first heard the tumor marker was back up. After receiving word from Saul, we became a bit more optimistic again. We just had to wait until the next blood test. It remained a constant battle.

I informed Wayne about what was going on. I also let him know that I had started work again and that I would not be home for Benjamin all day long, which meant that I could not always remind Benjamin to do things. I asked Wayne to make sure that Benjamin took action and made appointments when necessary. Someone needed to motivate him to do so, or sometimes actually make the appointments for him. We could not just sit back and wait for Benjamin to do so. The past had taught us that Benjamin was at times too relaxed about such things, or so it seemed, and that he needed guidance. On the other hand, I had discussed the situation with Benjamin, and we had come to an agreement that from now on I would not hassle him. I would not get all worked up when he decided to approach things in a different way than many other people would. He promised to ask me when he needed my help. If he did not ask for anything, I would not do anything, apart from preparing the sauna for him each day, preparing the apricot seeds, and helping him clean and bandage the wound on his back.

Wayne promised me he would keep an eye on Benjamin while I was out at work. He let me know that he had received Benjamin's national health insurance registration card along with the policy. It turned out that the local police department had assisted Benjamin by writing a letter that enabled him to register with social services. Once he was registered with social services, it was easy to obtain national health insurance. That was one less worry: Benjamin was now covered. Blue Cross had dropped Benjamin in January because he turned twenty-three beginning of February. Any reason Blue Cross could get to kick him out and not having to pay his medical bills any longer. But I was

---

harmful and abnormal immune complexes that precipitate autoimmune diseases, for example.

not finished with Blue Cross yet; I still was waiting to hear from them about my appeal. I had not accepted the 80 percent ruling.

The job in Sassenheim did not work out for me. I had forgotten about the awful traffic in Holland: traffic jams in the morning and traffic jams in the evening. It took me two hours both ways, regardless of whether I left early or late. I could not stand it. I informed the recruiter that I did not think I was willing to do this, but they begged me to try it for another week or so. I gave in and did. But no matter what time I went to work, traffic was just hopeless. After two weeks I let them know that this was not for me and that I was not coming in anymore. So from mid-February on, I was back at home again.

Life went on as before. I e-mailed friends and family in the United States to keep them updated on Benjamin. Everybody was sad to hear that his AFP tumor marker had gone up; they were worried. I also received word from my previous employer, IMG Americas. They were contacting me again, wondering whether if there was any way I would be willing to travel to the United States for at least a week for a blueprint and interview session with a client in California. Perhaps afterward, would I be willing to travel for a five-month period to the United States? They wanted me back, not necessarily as a full-time employee but perhaps as a freelance consultant. They were going to call me during the week of February 26, 2001. Because the job in Sassenheim had not worked out, I was considering IMG's proposal. I needed to wait and see what was proposed during our planned phone call.

If we had not had enough sad news, more was coming our way. Zoë and Frido broke up. She had left Frido the previous Monday and was staying with a girlfriend in Amsterdam. I did not know whether the separation was permanent or not. I had only spoken to Zoë briefly. She had to find a full-time job so that she could support herself. Until now she had worked part-time because she was busy trying to start a business herself. Another dream went out of the window—starting a business was not an option right now. I did not know what had happened. Normally when they had a fight Frido called me. He always wanted to discuss their differences with me. This time he had not done so; I had not heard a thing from him.

Then came more bad news. Toward the end of February I received a letter from Blue Cross that my appeal had been declined. The letter was dated January 23, but it had not arrived in Holland before because it had been sent to my old address in Austin before it finally made it to my address in Amersfoort. I was furious. The reason they gave was total nonsense. They said: "The Committee noted that while the treatment you received while abroad was required, ample time was provided in order to arrange transportation and receive treatment in the United States." What ample time? And it was not me who received treatment but my son Benjamin. I decided to react to their denial and let them know how I felt and what I thought about Blue Cross. I tried to call, without success. I left a voice mail asking for them to return my call, which they never did. So again I e-mailed them, just like before, when I tried to get my claims reimbursed. I explained that Benjamin had been in such condition that he could no longer walk, sit up, or sleep. No airline company would have allowed him on their plane. No airliner would fly him across the ocean. Did they really think I would have given up my house, my job, my life—my everything—in the United States to move over here if I thought he would be able to fly back to the States? I asked them if they had ever seen pictures of concentration camp victims from the Second World War. Well, that was how my son had looked like, just a bag of bones, and they were telling me he could have arranged transportation? Benjamin was very lucky to be alive. And he was only alive because he was admitted into the hospital in Amsterdam. He would have been dead, if he had had to fly back to the United States.

It is really sad that insurance companies think only of their shareholders rather than the well-being of their clients. I wrote that I hoped that the person who had denied my appeal would never be in a position where his or her child was dying of cancer and then he or she had to fight for the bills to be paid. "Let me assure you, the nightmare, the emotional rollercoaster, the turning upside down of your life that cancer causes are more than enough for anybody to handle. Having to fight to get your medical bills paid should not be part of it," I wrote. Last but not least I wanted to know if an insurance company could deny further coverage because a patient turned twenty-three years old, although his treatment was not yet finished. Of course I never received a reply. Nor did I bother anymore, as Benjamin was now covered by the Dutch system. This is exactly what those insurance companies want. They want you to give up in the end so that they don't have to pay you. At the time I did not have the energy or the desire to go after them, but I really should have sued them.

After my phone call with IMG Americas, I let them know that I was interested in the position they were offering but that I would prefer to work as a contractor. I had looked up the rates and discovered that in the United States they paid anywhere from $70 to $130 per hour. Here in Holland they paid pretty much the same per hour. I also told them that I would only travel business class now when I needed to travel overseas. I required access from home so that when possible I could work remotely rather than at the client in the United States. I needed to know as soon as possible about their decision, because if the offer did not go through, I needed to start looking for jobs here also. And that's exactly what I did; I started applying for jobs in Holland. Several companies invited me for an interview, and a couple of them offered me a job. However, the salary offered was way below my expectations, and I was not convinced the jobs were right for me. As a matter of fact, I still did not really know what I wanted. I was here in the Netherlands with mixed feelings, but I realized that for Benjamin's sake it was best, as no insurance company in the United States was going to insure him now.

The company I had worked for the previous month was not willing to pay for my services, because they felt I had no right to walk out after two weeks. I had provided them with the work they had requested, and I had a contract that stated that within the first month I could terminate without notice. But it was another set back. The year 2001 had not started very well. Too many bad things already happened in such a short period of time. It was almost spring, and I sincerely hoped that the remainder of the year would be better.

Things did brighten up a bit in March. Family and friends from abroad visited: Ken, my stepson; Amanda, Mike's niece; and Luc, a Swedish kid who had stayed with us in Austin as a foreign exchange student years earlier. We did not have enough spare rooms to put them up, but that did not matter to them. They were all young and willing to settle in the living room, either on an inflatable bed or on the couch.

They stayed for a week, and we enjoyed their company and had a good time. We showed them Amsterdam and took them out to different kind of restaurants. Benjamin took them out to one of those enormous house parties in Amsterdam, an all-night thing with hundreds of people. Benjamin was glad to see Ken again. He and his stepbrother had shared an apartment in Austin when they first stepped out into the world by themselves. They liked to play board games, such as chess. Amanda and Benjamin, although they had never met before, got on well with each other. They spent quite some time together discussing all sorts of things. Amanda had never been to Europe and had never flown before. She enjoyed the visit tremendously and later, when she was back home again, let me know that she was a little sad to be home again. Holland had won her heart over. It was quite different from the very small Texas town in the middle of nowhere where she came from. She hoped she would be able to come back soon.

Despite the little hiccups over the past months, we were all well. Life just carried on. On March 19, Zoë and Benjamin had gone to visit their little sister Sarah, who lived with her mother in Amsterdam and was celebrating her fifth birthday. Benjamin had another appointment scheduled for Tuesday, March 27, with his oncologist. I prayed to God that his tumor markers were going to be okay. Benjamin was still in good spirits, trying to look ahead and get on with his life. He went to an open house at a college he was interested in. Classes there would start in the fall. I was still not working; IMG Americas had not let me know one way or the other whether they would need me for the project in California. Apparently they were still waiting to hear from the client whether they had won the project.

In the beginning of April we received the blood test results. Again, the news was not good. The AFP marker had risen, this time from twenty to ninety-five. The other two tumor markers (beta HCG and LDH) were fine, both under five. I was very worried. I wondered whether it would be better for Benjamin to have the testicle removed. Perhaps that was causing the problem. The wound on his back was no longer discharging tissue, but it was still releasing fluid. I thought perhaps all the very enlarged lymph nodes in his abdomen and in his neck were trying to clean themselves up. I contacted all my medical friends and asked for answers yet again. Why did nobody know the answers?

Neither the conventional oncologists nor the holistic doctors could give me any definite answers. It seemed they were guessing just as much as I was. This awful disease was turning my life upside down again, and all I could do was live with it. It was becoming a familiar nightmare.

I didn't know how Benjamin felt about the increase in the AFP. He did not really open up to me and stayed very much to himself. Was he hiding? Did he not want to know? Or was he desperate? Did he believe what Dr. Levit, the oncologist in the United States, had told us: that the rising AFP could be because the existing tumor tissue was breaking down? On the other hand, it could also mean the growth of new tumor. He told us that if it seemed as if the immune response was taking care of the tumor, then all Benjamin had to do was reduce the amount of tumor tissue to a small enough quantity that his immune system could complete the job. What the hell did that mean?

Dr. Hoekman was convinced that the cancer was coming back and the increase meant more tumor growth. Benjamin had said a while back that he could feel three tumors in his lower body, but recently he could only feel one. He also mentioned that the tumor in his groin felt softer. The testicle itself was not causing any problems, but it had not shrunk. Benjamin was still feeling fine; he was in good spirits, despite the increase in AFP. He was eating well, and he had no pain anywhere. He believed the tumor mass was shrinking because he could sit up straight; his spine was becoming straight again. What was I to think of all this? All these different opinions and *no one* really knowing what was going on or what we needed to do. It was driving me crazy. And each of the professionals we were working with—Dr. Hoekman, Saul, and the other oncologists—came up with different suggestions: chemo, CT scans, other medication, et cetera, et cetera. And Benjamin simply continued with his daily saunas, took his vitamins and supplements, and drank his Essiac tea.

I knew that Benjamin would not go for any more chemo, nor would he have a CT scan done. I wondered whether he would go for an ultrasound. I told him that if my thoughts were worth anything to him that I recommended that he go for an ultrasound to see whether the tumor masses throughout his body were increasing or decreasing. At least he would know for sure and he would not have to assume.

If there was an increase, if it were I, I would have the testicle removed. If the testicle was the cause, the tumor count should become normal within thirty days.

If the tumor count was not normal, then perhaps he should start again with Laetrile IVs. Meanwhile, I hoped he'd continue with the daily saunas, vitamins, apricot seeds, et cetera.

That was all I wanted to tell him. I knew that pressuring him did not work. Benjamin was Benjamin, and he would do it his way. I needed to keep the faith where Benjamin was concerned. The mere fact that he was still alive, that he was looking well again and feeling better, was a testament to the treatment he had decided to follow. It was best not to panic at this point. I just hoped and prayed Benjamin would be on guard and not procrastinate with treatment, whatever it was going to be.

Apart from worrying about Benjamin, I had to seriously look for a consultancy job; my money was almost gone. I did not actually want to go back to work. I would rather stay home and be a mother and a wife. But I realized I needed to earn a living. In truth I did not want to work for anyone anymore. But starting something for myself required a lot of energy and enthusiasm, which I did not have. Perhaps that was due to Benjamin's disease, not knowing whether he would beat this or whether we would be on this rollercoaster ride of ups and downs for a long time. It was emotionally draining. The only alternative to generate some income was to work as a consultant once more.

During the day I talked to several recruiting agents and spent lots of time on the phone with them. In the end I accepted a job for three months in Brussels. It meant I needed to travel again. The idea was that on Mondays I would drive down to Brussels, stay in a hotel, and return on Fridays to Amersfoort. There were no opportunities closer to home at that moment, and I could not afford to wait for something else. I was to start on April 8. I was not happy leaving Benjamin, even though Mike was with him and I knew Mike would make sure he ate and took his saunas. But it wasn't the same. A mother should take care of her son, not a stepdad. I contacted Benjamin's dad Wayne to ask him to stay in contact with Benjamin and give him moral support. I also wanted Wayne to talk to Benjamin and see if he could convince him to have an operation to remove the testicle, especially because Benjamin had complained to me recently of backaches. It was the same kind of pain he had last year, except this time it was on the left side of his lower back. It did not sound good, and I was troubled. He needed to see a doctor.

The job in Brussels was not too bad. It took me about two and half hours to get there, and the commute was not as dreadful as I had anticipated. The company was in the middle of implementing SAP, which was part of a global rollout. They were looking for Dutch-speaking trainers. The company had produced tons of standard training material, which was used globally. However, everything was in English. The company in Brussels wanted their users to be trained in Dutch. The users were all in their facility in Herentals, and the actual training was going to take place in that facility. Apart from me, who was going to be responsible for the training of the sales and distribution module, there were five other trainers for the other modules. We were located in a large empty office space, far too large for just a handful of people. I was going to spend most of my time there for a couple of months or so.

Although there was tons of work to do adjusting and translating training materials, I did think a lot about Benjamin in between. I would e-mail him regularly; he would respond to my e-mail address at this company. He also forwarded the recruiters' messages I kept receiving. He always announced himself as "… your private secretary with the following message …" Hardly ever did he mention how he was feeling or express concern.

But one weekend when I was at home, he let me know his neck tumor was bothering him and beginning to hurt. It had started five days or so before. Of course he had not mentioned it to anyone. He had spent a lot of time in bed for a couple of days because he did not feel well. I looked at it; the tumor was red on one side. I wondered whether it had become infected or if perhaps this tumor was ready to break open like the tumor on his back had done. Maybe that explained the elevated AFP tumor marker. It seemed bigger. Perhaps the increase in size caused the pain because the skin was now stretched.

I suggested calling Dr. Hoekman. Naturally, Benjamin did not want to see a doctor. Benjamin's theory was that the lymph system was beginning to work again and was getting rid of the stuff in his bloodstream. Was he looking for excuses and justification for not wanting to see a doctor? Why did he not want to know what went on I his body? I asked him how much he weighed now. He weighted sixty-nine kilos with his dressing gown on, down from seventy-one kilos without it. The weight loss might be because he was worrying and not eating properly, but to me it was an obvious sign. I could not just sit and let it be, and I decided to contact Wayne. I recommended that he call Hoekman for Benjamin.

Perhaps we needed another approach and should just make appointments for him. For some reason Benjamin did not take action when action was required. He was too relaxed, and he could not afford to be relaxed, not with this awful disease. Zoë and I suggested that Benjamin talk to some kind of therapist or psychologist to help him deal with the cancer. We all thought it would do him good to talk to a professional to express his feelings and worries.

Although my entire life more or less revolved around Benjamin's cancer, life did carry on, and normal things did happen in my household. Zoë and Frido had resolved their issues and were back together again. Mike and I received an invitation to a wedding in the United States. Sadly, I was unable to go because of my consultancy contract in Brussels. There was no way I could take off during that assignment. But Mike ended up attending the wedding. Zoë and her partner were planning a three-week vacation to Spain in June. They rented a large house with a couple of bedrooms near the beach, so we were thinking of visiting them for a couple of days. I was definitely hoping that Benjamin would go for a week or so. It would do him good; besides, he needed some sunshine. The weather in Holland was lousy, still too cold for the season, with far too much rain.

My birthday, May 9, came and went. I was at work in Brussels—no typical Dutch birthday celebration for me that year. I received a nice electronic birthday card from Benjamin. Mike was still in Casper and did not get back until May 13. I received a couple of e-mails from friends and relatives in the United States, among them an e-mail from my friend Moe, who was finally moving to San Diego from Austin to be with her sister Kathleen. Kathleen, a young woman in her mid-thirties, had been diagnosed with cancer about a year before Benjamin was diagnosed. Another friend and ex-colleague e-mailed me to let me know the latest news at my previous employer and how she was doing personally. It was good to hear from them all, and I missed them. How my life had changed in just a year and a half—it was turned totally upside down.

Benjamin had another appointment the end of May. I was praying that the tumor markers were stable and had not gone up again. He seemed okay again and said he felt okay. The neck tumor did not seem to bother him anymore. Maybe it had just been an infection. In the meantime Benjamin had invested in turntables and a mix panel. All this equipment was connected to his computer, and he was practicing DJ work. I was amazed the neighbors had not complained yet, with him playing music pretty loud almost the entire day. He had entered a competition for a two-week course at a music academy in New York. He said he wanted to be a DJ. At least he was keeping busy and focusing on something he enjoyed doing. Apparently there was big money to be earned if you were a good DJ.

In the beginning of June we received another blood test result. For the third time in a row, the result was not good. The AFP tumor marker had gone up again. It was now over five hundred. It appeared that the AFP was rising by a factor of five every two months. This was very worrying indeed. Benjamin's oncologist again recommended further rounds of chemo, but Benjamin refused that option. I would not be me if I did not do further research, and so again I was exploring the Internet. I looked at the Acor Web page.[48] It featured lots of relevant information on testicular cancer. I copied and pasted some text I found on that page and forwarded it to Benjamin, hoping that perhaps he would now reconsider the suggestion I had made a few months back to have his testicle removed.

Benjamin read the material and considered an operation; he discussed it with me, saying that it was probably the way to go. But he did not want just any urologist to remove the testicle. He absolutely did not want the operation done in the VU Hospital in Amsterdam, because Benjamin and the VU urologist did not connect very well. He questioned me about whether he should perhaps go back to the United States and have the operation there. He read somewhere about Dr.

48.   http://tcrc.acor.org/ The Testicular Cancer Resource Center

Foster from the Indiana University Hospital; apparently Dr. Foster was considered one of the best. I suggested that he contact Dr. Foster to see what the possibilities were, if any, to be operated on as soon as possible. Benjamin also needed to find out whether they would accept Dutch national health insurance, or whether perhaps they would be able to help free of charge because Benjamin's was such an extraordinary case. It could benefit their research. He also needed to check his insurance policy to see whether treatment abroad was covered. I suggested if going to the United States was out of the question, he start calling different Dutch testis urologists. Surely there were others who could perform the operation besides the one in the VU.

On June 8, 2001, Benjamin wrote an e-mail to Dr. Foster. He explained his situation from May 1999 until the present. He told Dr. Foster about his alternative treatments and how Laetrile had worked, but treatment had not shrunk his tumors, nor had they gotten any bigger while he had been on Laetrile. He reported that chemotherapy had also worked to bring down his tumor markers, but that did not shrink his tumors either. He wrote that he now felt he needed to have his testicle removed and wanted to know what the latest advances in surgery were. He believed Dr. Foster was the best in this field, and he wondered whether he was willing to do the surgery for Benjamin.

About five hours later the same day, Benjamin received a reply from Dr. Foster. I was always impressed how willing the United States doctors and specialists were to answer your e-mails or phone calls. Dr. Foster informed him that without seeing his films it was difficult to give an opinion. Residual disease in the abdomen should be removed along with the testicle. He knew of no "new" techniques for doing this. He suggested, however, that the surgeon should be experienced in testis cancer. The people in Europe he knew who had the most experience were Tim Christmas in England; Peter Albers in Bonn, Germany; Giorgio Pizzocaro in Italy; and Lothar Weissbach, also in Germany. He was sure there were other capable surgeons. He thought Benjamin should strongly consider surgery based upon what he had told him.

In the meantime, Benjamin learned that his insurance would not cover the operation abroad, because there were many urologists who could perform surgery here in Holland. We therefore stopped pursuing the option of having it done in the United States. I did not care where it was going to be performed. I was just happy that Benjamin had decided to have the tumor removed. I was almost sure that the testicle tumor was causing the increase in AFP.

Dr. Foster had recommended some good people in Europe, and because Benjamin was a British citizen on the weekend I was back from Brussels I decided to write my friend Mark from the Finchley Clinic to see if he could help out. Dr. Foster mentioned Dr. Tim Christmas, who supposedly worked in the Charing Cross Hospital, but I could not find anything on the Web about either the hospital or the doctor. I asked whether Mark could perhaps find out for me how I could reach the doctor. Perhaps he could get a telephone number, or an e-mail address? At the same time I let him know how Benjamin was doing and that his AFP tumor marker had been rising since the beginning of the year. At the same time I started researching Dutch urologists with experience in testis cancer. The Acor's Web site was once again a good reference site. It contained numerous names of specialists from hospitals all over the world. Whoever had taken the time to gather all that information and do all the research had done an excellent job.

I located a couple of the doctors who were recommended and decided to e-mail Dr. Mulders from the Academic Hospital in Nijmegen (Netherlands). I explained the situation and said that my son had lived in the United States, where no one looked down upon you when you asked doctors critical questions or when you asked for references, which was not normal in Holland. In the past Benjamin had been shouted at by doctors, offended that he dared to question them. This had caused distrust and the disturbed relationship with the urologist in the VU Hospital in Amsterdam. I explained that Benjamin did not want to be operated on by the VU urologist. I wrote that Benjamin was looking for an urologist whom he could work with, someone who would not pressure him into doing anything he did not want—someone who would listen and take his concerns seriously.

Mark came back to me with telephone numbers and the address of the Charing Cross Hospital in London. He could not give me any reference as to whether the hospital was a good one. However, Benjamin might get in fast if he went in as a private patient, which would be very expensive. If he wanted to do it through the National Health Service

(NHS), it would take some time. He urged Benjamin to have some electro-crystal therapy afterward to calm the site down. It would speed up the healing. He was sorry that the ozone had not cured Benjamin and was wondering what went wrong, because he had seen pictures of the tumor being discharged from his abdomen. Nothing had really gone wrong with the ozone. As we would find out later, there were many tumors in his body we did not know about and so we did not cup. The problem all along had been that none of the treatments had actually reduced the tumor mass in Benjamin's body. Neither the Laetrile IVs nor the chemotherapy did shrink any of his tumors.

I also received a reply from Dr. Peter Mulders, but not until four days later. He and another doctor, Professor de Mulder, both worked in the Academic Hospital in Nijmegen as medical oncologists specializing in urologic tumors. He gave me the telephone numbers where both of them could be reached should we desire to make an appointment. Dr. Mulders apologized for not responding earlier but he had just returned from the United States.

In the end Benjamin decided to have the operation done here in Holland, and he had made an appointment with the urologist in Nijmegen for June 13, 2001. Because the hospital needed Benjamin's x-rays, I had gone to the VU hospital personally to pick them up so that we could take them along with us to Nijmegen. This way we would not need the postal service to deliver them and wouldn't worry whether we'd receive them in time for the appointment. We finally saw all the x-rays that had been taken. Two-thirds of his abdomen was involved with tumor masses. Now we could see that none of that mass had decreased during the rounds of chemo.

The oncologist in Nijmegen told Benjamin the same thing as Dr. Foster had. He needed to have not only the testicle removed but also all the tumors in his abdomen. The oncologist did not think that more chemo would do any good. A CT scan and another blood test were done. Benjamin was expected to be back for the results on June 20.

A day after Benjamin's first appointment with the doctors in Nijmegen, we heard that Wayne, his father, was in the hospital. Benjamin went to visit him; apparently Wayne had experienced severe chest pains and as a precaution had gone to the hospital. Apart from us nobody knew Wayne was in the hospital. Zoë was still in Spain. I told

Benjamin he needed to inform his grandmother and his aunts that their son and brother was in the hospital and to let them know the phone number where he could be reached. God forbid that something awful happened.

Benjamin was scheduled to go into the hospital on Friday, June 29. He was expected around ten o'clock in the morning. I had arranged with my client that Thursday, June 28, would be my last day. I made sure that before then, the trainings I was conducting would last an hour a day longer so that I covered all the material that needed to be covered. I explained to my students why my last day was going to be Thursday. I liked working with the Belgian users. I found them very pleasant, willing, and not as arrogant and snobbish as the Dutch. They were very compassionate; when they found out about Benjamin, they were truly concerned and wished him best of luck.

The new CT scan was compared to the ones from the VU hospital, it was evident that one large tumor in his abdomen had cleared itself up. Of course we knew that, and we had the pictures of the wound discharging dead tumor tissue to prove it. However, the new CT scan also showed that other large tumors in his abdomen had taken its place. If Benjamin wanted the complete tumor mass to be removed, it would require an operation of twenty hours or more. During the operation he was going to need artificial blood vessels because his own blood vessels would likely be cut during the removal of the tumors. Benjamin needed to think about all this. We did receive one bit of good news: the AFP tumor marker had gone done slightly. His other tumor markers were still normal. We were told once again that further chemo would do no good. This contradicted what Dr. Hoekman from the VU hospital, who was in favor of more chemo, wanted. The doctor also suggested a PET scan. Apparently a PET scan can reveal active areas. For now Benjamin decided he was just going to have his testis removed.

As Friday, June 29, approached, Benjamin became nervous, although he tried hard not to let on. On Thursday evening we discussed the operation. It would be the first time in his life that Benjamin would undergo an operation, and he did not know what to expect. I explained my experience with the few operations I had and said that it was nothing to worry about it. "By the time you wake up, it is all over, without ever realizing what happened," I told him. He asked me to promise him that once this was behind him and he had survived it that I'd go with him to the gym on a regular basis. He wanted to get fit and start building some muscle. I believe around this time that Benjamin had met a girl he was rather fond of. Her name was Emmelien. As a matter of fact, I believe he was about to fall in love with her. He talked about her to me, and that was enough for me to realize he was in love, because normally he did not discuss girlfriends at all. I was extremely happy for him. Having a dear person in his life would help him not think about this awful disease all the time. It could lift some of the heavy burden from his shoulders.

I dropped Benjamin off on Friday morning and drove back home. In the afternoon I returned to visit him. He was back in his room and doing fine. He was out of the anesthesia and feeling okay. During the evening I went back to visit him again, together with Mike. Benjamin seemed relieved and did not experience anything negative from the operation. He felt at peace and wondered why he had not had it done before. But Benjamin's dilemma had always been that he thought too much about everything. He analyzed and constantly asked himself questions about the right thing to do. He also looked at everything that could go wrong and at the complications. Most people don't think; they just trust and do it.

Saturday morning, June 30, I returned to pick him up again. The whole ordeal had not been too bad. We were told the mass encapsulating the tumor was a mature teratoma[49] with mostly fluid. The testis tumor itself apparently was a mature teratoma within a mature teratoma, and a yolk sac tumor (a malignant germ cell neoplasm) was still active. The doctor also suspected further cancer activity within the tumors in his abdomen. Regardless, Benjamin felt good and self-assured. He had lost a lot of weight though, I think mainly because of his worries about the operation. He had barely eaten at all lately and during the one-night stay in the hospital he had not eaten at all. But now that he was back home his appetite was coming back; as soon as he started eating, his weight increased again. He was ready to move on with his life and leave everything behind him. Now that the testicular tumor was gone, he

---

49.   A type of benign (noncancerous) germ cell tumor, a type of tumor that begins in the cells that give rise to sperm or egg, that often contains several different types of tissue, such as hair, muscle, and bone. Also called a dermoid cyst.

felt he had conquered the disease and that the tumor markers would continue to decrease. We were expected back at the Academic Hospital for a follow-up visit on Wednesday, July 11. Surely the doctors would want to discuss with Benjamin what he was going to do about the abdominal tumor mass. Did he want to go for the operation; would he go for a PET scan—what would the next steps be?

I decided that before we returned to the hospital, I'd check with my friend Dr. Levit in the States to see what his opinion was. I also updated my holistic friend in Canada. There was no harm in getting people's opinion. I asked them if they knew of a way to get rid of the tumor mass without surgery. Dr. Levit replied that he did not know of a way other than surgery, unless the tumor was susceptible to one of the new treatments like anti-angiogenesis factor. [50] He also mentioned not to be surprised if the AFP level did not go down for six weeks. It sometimes took a while for tumor factors to clear the body. On the other hand, he said, if AFP was being produced by the neck masses, then the numbers would not go down at all. He did not recommend abdominal surgery unless Benjamin was forced into it because of obstruction. Even with the most meticulous surgery it was difficult to remove all the tumor mass, especially if more tissue remained elsewhere in the body. It was possible that someone was using antibodies directly against AFP as a therapeutic approach, which might be of benefit to Benjamin. He asked whether Benjamin's health insurance would cover Benjamin in one of the United States hospitals, perhaps the National Institutes of Health or even the University of Chicago. Benjamin's case was quite unusual, and Dr. Levit felt it might be of interest to some researchers there in the United States. Dr. Levit was also interested in seeing the pathology report of the most recent neck biopsy. Both neck tumor biopsies—the one in the United States and the one in Amsterdam—showed it was not cancer. But what was it? Nobody seemed to be able to answer that question, not to me anyway.

Saul replied to let me know he was surprised to hear of the extensive growth of the tumor in the abdomen. The fluid was a concern as well, and he stressed the fact that that needed to be drained. All he could advise for now was to continue with the ozone saunas and to funnel over the abdomen where the tumors were, plus the neck and back. He also

---

50.   Angiogenesis: the growth of new blood vessels.

recommended a liver cleanse; he could not remember whether he ever mentioned it, but it certainly was an important part of the protocol.

Dr. Levit then said if the tumor in the abdomen had a collection of fluid which could be conveniently drained, it would be worth trying. If the tumor was like a sponge, with many small pockets of fluid, then drainage was not possible. He also asked if Benjamin's oncologist thought that any therapy instilled intra-abdominally would be of value. Of course I did not know what that meant. Apparently this therapy involved having a needle inserted into the peritoneal cavity to evacuate as much fluid as possible. Then a solution of chemotherapy drug is injected into the abdomen, and the patient is rolled around to allow the chemo to make contact with as much of the tumor as possible. Since it was not injected intravenously, the patient had essentially no side effects, and the medication went exactly where it should go. Apparently this therapy was used for ovarian cancer patients. It seemed to make sense to me. But if this was a possibility, would Benjamin accept a chemo-related therapy?

I forwarded all the information I received from my global friends to Benjamin. I never pushed him one way or the other anymore. I knew from my past struggles that that did not work. It was best to provide him with the information and to let him make up his mind one way or the other. After all he was an adult, and no one could make him do anything. He was in charge; it was his life, regardless of how much I worried about him—and I was worried again, especially after he mentioned that just recently he was experiencing pains in his hip.

One of the chemotherapy side effects Benjamin experienced was that any little wound or infection on his hands or feet did not seem to heal. Benjamin had some kind of infection on his feet that did not want to go away. I was not sure what it was, whether it was athlete's foot or some other infection. Antifungal creams and sprays did not work. In the end I suggested he take a footbath on a daily basis with some drops of tea tree oil in it and that during the day he put some drops of the oil on the infection. Within weeks the infection cleared up, and his feet started to heal.

I had hoped that I would be at home for a while once my contract in Brussels ended. But that did not happen. Almost immediately after

I finished in Brussels, I was assigned another project in The Hague. I had a brief interview with the project manager of the company in The Hague; they wanted me to start as early as Wednesday, July 4, 2001. There seemed no time to relax.

I commuted daily back and forth from Amersfoort to The Hague. Although normally it should take not more than fifty minutes each way, I soon found out that I got stuck in traffic daily; actual travel time was two hours there and two hours back each day. Every day was awful. I checked whether there was a possibility I could use public transportation. In the past, I remembered, public transportation had always been very good and very reliable, but I had not used it for years and definitely not since I had been back in Holland. I was fortunate; there was a direct train from Amersfoort via Utrecht to The Hague. No need to switch trains; I could stay put all the way.

An advantage of being a freelance consultant was that whenever you needed to take care of private matters, you took the time you needed and let the company know what hours you would be out of the office. It worked well for me, especially because I did need a lot of time to drive Benjamin to his appointments.

The month of July went by without too many hiccups. Benjamin had gone back to the Academic Hospital in Nijmegen for follow-up appointments. During one of those appointments the doctors told Benjamin that a 20-hour or so operation was not without risk. They were almost sure Benjamin would end up with a catheter in his side, and the chances that he would end up in a wheelchair for the rest of his life were real. This was because artificial vessels needed to be used during the operation. And there was no guarantee that surgeons could successfully remove the entire tumor mass. The oncologist also told Benjamin that he would not grow old with that tumor mass. Benjamin remained pretty calm, and the information did not seem to worry him too much. We discussed it a bit, not at great length, and Benjamin said that ending up in a wheelchair was no option for him. He decided not to have the operation.

Life continued almost normally. Benjamin practicing his DJ work, trying to perfect his mixing skills. According to Benjamin, mixing was more than just pasting two records together. It meant harmonizing two otherwise separate sources of sound. He also continued socializing and hanging out with his new girlfriend. I continued working for a living, getting frustrated in traffic jams when I did not use public transportation or getting frustrated when I did use the train and ended up in the middle of nowhere, because the rail managers were once again causing all sorts of problems. Ever since public transportation had gone private and was no longer run by the government, the service and efficiency had totally gone out of the window. I was also getting very frustrated with, or rather envious of, Mike. There he was, at home, making no effort at all to try to find a job and work for a living. I resented the fact that he did not attempt to find a job and help me share the load equally.

Zoë was working for a fashion company; once in a while she had to travel abroad. In the beginning of August she was required to go to Copenhagen, Denmark, and she asked whether I felt like accompanying her on the trip. She said she would love it if I came along. During the past year and a half I had barely spent any time alone with Zoë, and I felt it would be nice to go with her. I checked whether I could arrange a cheap flight on short notice. Low fares required booking at least three days in advance, so I did not qualify. I had to pay full price and fly business class rather than economy. I did not mind, but Zoë was booked in economy class. It meant we would just have to sit separately during the short flight. Copenhagen was only one and a half hours away, so we would endure. But the cabin crew had a pleasant surprise when we flew to Copenhagen on August 11, 2001. They let Zoë travel in business class as well. We sat in the front of the plane next to each other.

We had a smooth flight, and before we knew it we had touched down in Copenhagen. The hotel was in the center of Copenhagen, within walking distance of the stores and restaurants. During the day we visited the Fashion Fair and looked at the upcoming fashion styles. We enjoyed dinner together and a bit of shopping in the center of Copenhagen. The two-day visit was enjoyable, and I was glad I had taken the opportunity to get away for a short break. I thought I should really consider doing so more often.

The following Monday I was back working in The Hague, back in my daily routine of getting up early, taking the train from Amersfoort to The Hague, returning around 6:00 PM. It was almost boring; there was not much excitement going on. Mike and Benjamin were both at home doing their thing, whatever it was that kept them busy all day. Benjamin was happy, though; he felt that he had conquered his cancer. Because Benjamin was so happy and cancer was not really mentioned anymore, we all accepted that he had beaten the disease. In retrospect we, especially I, should have known better. But the medical professionals hadn't told us that the tumors were ticking time bombs. And we all needed a break from the constant worry, and Benjamin's happiness allowed that. We tried to live a normal life without the burden of cancer on our minds all the time.

Benjamin was very happy; I now know he was deeply in love at that time. He wanted to forget about his disease and be a happy young man, a young man who enjoyed life. After the operation his AFP tumor markers had dropped from nine hundred to three hundred: still not perfect by any means, but the markers were at least dropping again. The stuff left in his body was like a ghost town, Benjamin said, vacant and empty.

He got out more and spent more time with his father, who was now out of the hospital, trying to bond and build a relationship once again. Benjamin had joined a local sports club and was also thinking of going to Crete for a vacation. He was getting back to his old self again, the Benjamin we knew before.

After his operation Benjamin was so sure that he had beaten the cancer, that any tumors still in his body were now just dead tissue, that he no longer took daily ozone saunas. I don't know what made him believe that he had crushed the cancer. Maybe it was possible because he was in love and optimistic about everything. But I now know that when dealing with cancer there is no room for being off-guard, no room for letting up on treatment. However, that was exactly what Benjamin did. And so did I. We wanted to believe he had recovered and that we could live "normal" lives, whatever normal is.

Then, out of the blue, on Monday, August 27, 2001, I received an e-mail from my husband, Mike. Mike and I lived together, yet he sent me an e-mail. He felt that our relationship had deteriorated, that it was not right and had not been for the last few years. It was a very long e-mail. He wrote that he, too, felt that Benjamin was now on the mend and that he was no longer needed. He had been here to support us and had been a companion and a friend. But now it was time to leave; his goal was to rebuild his relationship with his sons. He wanted to help them to reach their full potential.

I was flabbergasted. That's all I needed! A stupid e-mail from my husband telling me he was leaving me. Why could not he just talk to me, communicate his problems and concerns? And his brainless excuse of wanting to be there for his sons … His sons were twenty-four and twenty-six years old. They were living their own lives; they had made their choices, and they were definitely not waiting for their father to start interfering with their lives. It was too absurd for words. I was so furious that I sent him a very short e-mail back, telling him that I had nothing to say and that I wanted him out of the apartment within a few days. And that's what he did. The next day when I came back from work he was gone. No note, no good-bye, nothing. I had no idea where he was, whether he had already left Holland, whether he was on a plane to Austin, or what. I could not believe he would just leave like that, without a word. It made me feel sick. I certainly didn't need another worry on top of all the stress and emotional aches and pains I had endured over the past two years. How easy for him to just walk away and not to take any responsibilities for anything. All his belongings were still here. We were still married. Did he expect that I would just take on all this additional work, pack up his stuff, and ship it back to the United States? That I would take care of the divorce and all the legal issues that follow?

Then I found a note to his son on his computer, in which he wrote that someday he might find a way to talk to me about his thoughts and feelings, but not right now. How could he be so cruel? Who can you talk to, who can you confide in, if not your partner? I did realize that our relationship had not been optimal, but what did he expect when I had to deal with an awful disease like cancer? On top of that, I always had been and still was the breadwinner: I always took charge and was responsible. Tons of burdens, worries, and concerns rested on my shoulders. Mike's mere presence, him saying "I love you," were not enough. I needed someone who shared the load with me, in all respects. I needed someone who understood my frustrations, who saw my loneliness, who communicated with me and shared his concerns. Mike did not do those things. Yes, he was right. Our relationship was not right, by any means.

The first couple of days after he left were awful. I tried to continue with my life as I had always done. Thank god I had a demanding job and tons of stuff on my mind. That did help some, but not enough to take away all the pain and heartache. I lost about eight pounds the first week he was gone. At least his leaving had been good for something. Benjamin typed up a letter on his computer to say that he would be there for me, especially if I needed someone to talk to. I am not sure how he felt about it all, but I don't think he was too sorry that Mike had left. He got on with Mike okay, and the two of them joked with each other once in a while, but that was about it. Benjamin felt more relaxed without Mike.

Toward the end of August I drove Benjamin to the hospital in Nijmegen for another blood test. This was the last one he would have in Nijmegen. His AFP marker had gone down again, but only slightly. His oncologist said that it might never totally go down. The other two markers were normal and had been normal since he finished chemotherapy. Benjamin was in good spirits those days. He decided not to go for monthly blood checks anymore, because it would make no difference, as he would not take additional chemo treatments. I did not agree with his decision, but Benjamin was Benjamin. He was an adult and responsible for his own actions.

After Mike left I started updating my relatives and friends in the States on how we were doing. Susan told me that Jason and Amy, her son and his fiancé, had bought a house and were going to get married at the beginning of the coming year. She knew all our names were on the guest list, and she said how wonderful it would be if we could all come over for the wedding. Yes, I thought, it would be nice to see them all. I hoped everyone on this side of the ocean was interested in going.

Susan and I also shared e-mails back and forth. I explained that Mike and I had broken up. We discussed relationships at length, and I was glad I had someone I could express my frustrations to. I had been deeply hurt and needed someone to talk to. Susan was a true friend. She was always there for me; she listened to my problems and responded immediately to my e-mails. It helped to get it off my chest. It also allowed me to start thinking about my relationship with Mike and what it was I really wanted. Would I be willing to go back to the

United States? Mike was a true Texan; he had never felt at home in Holland and never successfully integrated. I did not think that would ever change.

Finally, after more than a week, I received word from Mike that he was staying with his son Ken in Austin. We started writing lengthy e-mails to each other, about how we felt and what was wrong. We were both sorry that we never tried to solve our problems and that we did not really understand each other. On paper we were able to express our thoughts and feelings. Now that we were thousands of miles apart, we were finally communicating. It was ridiculous! Why could not we do so when we were together? After weeks of e-mailing and talking on the phone for hours, we decided we wanted to give the relationship another chance and agreed we were both willing to work on it with professional help.

On September 11, 2001, during the afternoon, I received a phone call at work from Benjamin. He was in the gym and had been working out. After his workout, he had watched CNN on the TV screens that hung in the gym and had seen the news. Terrorists had attacked the United States. Airplanes had flown into the World Trade Center buildings in New York, the same buildings Benjamin and I had visited when we were in New York two years earlier, when we had returned from Dr. Schachter's clinic. What devastating news. In the meantime, my co-workers had also learned about the tragedy, and it became the discussion of the day. I could no longer concentrate and decided to leave and go home.

In the past I had had bad dreams about wars; I dreamed that Mike and I got separated and were unable to get back together because of tragedies like this. I was just hoping that Bush could keep his cool and not do anything stupid to make things worse. What would all this mean for Mike's planned flight back? Would he still be able to come back to Holland?

Europeans were shocked by what had happened in the States and felt very united with the Americans. September 14 became a day of mourning in Europe; at twelve o'clock we observed a three-minute silence to remember those killed during the tragedy. Concerts and dinners were organized to raise money for the victims, but apart from that life continued more or less as before here in Europe.

Perhaps it was all the stress and my problems with Mike, but during this period I did not feel very well. My back ached, I had a bad throat, and I was losing my voice. I needed to relax and try not to worry too much. But without Mike, relaxing and taking it easy were difficult. My days were long, and I was tired. Normally I would get up around 6:00 AM so that I could catch the 7:10 bus to the train station and arrive at work around 8:45 AM. I usually left work just before 5:00 PM and got back to the house around 6:30 PM. Mike had normally done all the housework, and he cooked every night. I needed to do all those chores now. Benjamin did help out by cleaning up, and occasionally he cooked. I missed Mike and could not wait for him to get back.

Mike had returned in October, and we slowly tried to work on our relationship. In light of the terrorist attack the previous month, Susan wondered whether we were still considering coming to Jason's wedding in February. Benjamin seemed to be doing fine. His last blood results didn't seem to interest him, so I did not know whether the tumors were now all benign, or whether we should still worry. Benjamin said it did not make any difference, and he seemed to be happy not knowing. He was still very much in love with Emmelien.

Benjamin was seeing some kind of therapist. He did not talk about it, but he went to see the man weekly. I was glad for him. At last it seemed he was dealing with his feelings and letting them out. He was in good spirits and never complained. I admired him for that. Living in Holland was a blessing for Benjamin. Here he was covered by the national health system, and I no longer had to pay enormous amounts of money for his treatments. Benjamin received a nice allowance from the Dutch government every month, which allowed him to take care of himself financially. He had purchased a digital camera and recording, editing, and mixing equipment and was busy making music. He had his own Web site, and listeners could even hear his music through his site. He kept himself busy during the day with his music; in the evenings he went out with friends and socialized with his peers.

Mike's oldest son, John, and his wife, Chantel, who lived in Montana, were expecting their second child in January, and I was busy ordering bits and pieces online for the new baby. I also spent time e-mailing friends and relatives in the United States. My sister-in-law Paula, who had worked in the travel industry, lost her job due to September 11. I e-mailed my friend Moe. She had recently moved to San Diego, California, to be with her sister who had been diagnosed with breast cancer approximately a year before Benjamin was diagnosed. She was now working 100 percent remotely. Her employer was in Austin. Her sister Kathleen was still hanging on, although she had stage four cancer. She was trying a new clinical trial chemo and an anti-cancer drug. So many people had cancer, it seemed—so many victims and so few survivors.

I was still reading any and all articles on cancer that came across my path. I forwarded them all to Benjamin. One of theses articles was particularly interesting. It discussed a newly developed molecule that starved cancer cells and made tumors vanish. This molecule, called *icon,* was able to kill the cells that make up the tumor's blood vessels and thus starve the tumor. But this new development had only been tested on mice. Researches were seeking FDA approval to use icon in humans. It might still take years before we understood whether that entirely new development would work in humans.

In the beginning of December Benjamin told me that he was looking for a place of his own. He felt it was time to start living by himself again. He and Mike never really got on that well, and Benjamin would rather have his own place. I was not pleased about that, because I was sure he was not yet ready to do so. He still needed someone to make sure he ate three proper meals a day and to assist him whenever assistance was needed. He needed a certain daily routine, and living by himself, I knew, he would not follow that routine. But I could understand his reasoning and his desire to move out. Besides, our current apartment was rather small for the three of us. We could all do with a bit more space. So I concluded that perhaps it was time I started looking for something more suitable, somewhere Benjamin could have more space and be more by himself but where I would still be nearby and could keep an eye on him when necessary.

I found the perfect place in Diemen, a small town next to Amsterdam, the town where Zoë lived with her partner Frido. The house I found was three stories high. The ground floor was about seven hundred square feet, a large space with a small hall, a small kitchen, and a bathroom. It had its own front door and would be perfect for Benjamin. The space was four to five times larger than his bedroom in our apartment. From the hall a door opened onto another hallway that led to the staircase for the other two floors. This hallway had another front door. In other words, the house had two front doors, one for the ground floor and one for the second and third floors. The second floor contained two very large bedrooms, a landing, and a large bathroom. The third floor contained the living room, dining room and kitchen, plus a half bath and a very large balcony. The house was available for rent as of March 1, 2002. We were all very enthusiastic about the house, including Benjamin. The downstairs could easily be split into a living area and a sleeping area. It was self-contained and ideal for Benjamin. If he wanted to entertain friends, they did not need to come through our part of the house, because we would both have our own front door. Benjamin could just come upstairs via the hallway door. He could still enjoy dinner with us should he desire. In case he needed medical attention or any help, all I had to do was to go down the stairs through the hallway into his "apartment."

The rent was high, but I earned enough to be able to afford the place, and both Benjamin and Mike were going to chip in. I decided to sign the rental agreement. We now had something to look forward to, and we had a couple of months to get the place in order. Benjamin's ground floor needed carpet and curtains; the bathroom and kitchen needed updating, and of course he needed furniture to decorate the place and to make it his home.

Christmas approached. The previous year we had celebrated at home with the family and Kathleen, Benjamin's friend from Texas. Mike's sons had not been with us, and I knew Mike missed them, especially around this time of the year. The problem was that Mike's sons never seemed to have enough vacation time to take a week or two off to come over. Therefore, I sought alternatives. When Benjamin was in the hospital we had dreamed of all going on a summer holiday once he was discharged. That never happened, mainly because Mike and I had to return to the United States twice that year. And that summer Benjamin had still been very weak and unable to walk far. His back had bothered him a lot, and he had been most comfortable just lying down. During

2001 when Benjamin did feel much better, we had not made plans for a fun vacation.

So I wondered if, instead of celebrating Christmas in Holland, we could all get together at a ski resort somewhere in North America, so that Mike's sons could join us for a few days. I was looking into places in Montana and in Canada. I saw some beautiful cabins for twelve or more persons. I asked Benjamin what he thought about the idea, and he thought it was great. He would love to go and ski. Mike was a bit hesitant because of the cost involved. But I felt that now that I was earning a substantial income as a freelance consultant, this was a once-in-a-lifetime opportunity. If we did not go for it now, who knows when I would be able to afford such a vacation again, especially because we would be moving in a couple of months to a far more expensive place. We needed to go for it now. I was all excited about it and started looking into what it would take to make this happen.

But then around mid-December, Benjamin's appetite started to decrease. He felt unwell, and he tired very quickly. He spent more time in bed than he usually did. I worried about him. He complained about backaches; he thought perhaps the pain came from him sitting behind turntables and mixing equipment all day long. It seemed wise to wait until Benjamin felt better before making vacation arrangements. In the end no arrangements were made, and instead we celebrated Christmas once again in our small two-bedroom apartment in Amersfoort.

In Holland we celebrate two days of Christmas, December 25 and 26. The second Christmas day, Benjamin celebrated at Klaas and Mariska's, but he came home rather early because of back pains and feeling unwell. I was not sure what to think of it all. I did not know how Benjamin felt through all this, but for me it was hell having to cope with the chronic uncertainty of his health. I worried more than Benjamin, and yet I was not the one with this awful disease. Did I need to start worrying again? I felt I would leave it for now and wait until the New Year before taking any action. It was almost the end of 2001, and Zoë's birthday was coming up.

CHAPTER 7

The Beginning

Dedicated to my only friend
He who will be there for me in the end
He who will take my pain away
On my final day
He who I can always count on
Even after I am gone.
Death ...

Benjamin Hyman

We celebrated Zoë's twenty-sixth birthday party at a disco bar in Hilversum. Benjamin and his friend Klaas were responsible for the music. They were experts now at mixing music, and both had their own mixing tables. Benjamin had been practicing for weeks, making sure he was the best. I know he was nervous, as this was his first time that he would be performing for a large audience. But there was no need to be nervous; he had everything under control, and the music he mixed sounded perfect. Looking at him standing there behind the turntables made me proud. However, I suddenly realized how thin and pale he looked. I knew over the past couple of weeks he had been experiencing bad backaches again, and I had advised him to go and see a chiropractor to learn what was causing the backaches. I didn't realize it might be the cancer playing up again. Benjamin didn't complain about his pains and aches much to me, because he did not want to worry me, so I did not often know what was going on. I talked to his best friends, Klaas and Mariska, to see if he had confided in them. Benjamin had spent Christmas with them just a week earlier, and Mariska had also noticed that he was losing weight again. However, when she asked to discuss the matter, Benjamin had refused.

I made up my mind at that moment. If he was not going to do anything about it, I would. The next day, on December 31, I called our family doctor, Dr. Schellart, and asked if he would write out a referral note so that Benjamin could have his blood checked. He was a bit hesitant because he was only a family doctor and not very familiar with cancer. I said I would contact the oncologist to forward him the necessary details, so that Benjamin could have his blood checked at the local hospital rather than having to drive all the way to Amsterdam or Nijmegen. I also made an appointment for him at the chiropractor. The appointment was for January 21, 2002, at 8:00 AM. It seemed a long wait, but the assistant assured me that normally chiropractors have a waiting list of months rather than weeks. So I did not complain.

I forwarded the details via e-mail to Benjamin. I normally communicated via e-mail when I wanted to get some facts across so that he would remember and not forget. I also told Benjamin that I had asked our family doctor for a referral note. Later I found out the doctor had talked to Benjamin on the phone and said he was not able, or rather not willing, to write the note. I was not at home when the doctor called, but I did not like it one bit. How ridiculous! Why should we have to drive all the way to Nijmegen for a simple blood test that could be done anywhere? So I e-mailed Dr. Schellart and gave him the phone number and e-mail address of Benjamin's oncologist, asking him to contact him to ask what values needed to be tested. How difficult was that? I assured him that he did not need to be able to read or understand the results. Dr. Witjes, the oncologist in Nijmegen, would interpret them. We just needed to know the numbers, to assess the current situation and learn whether the cancer was progressing.

I just could not sit and wait until the appointment for blood tests. I felt I had to take charge and do anything I could to help Benjamin. I contacted the Cerbe organization in Canada. In 2000 I had ordered the 714X therapy, which Benjamin had never used. The unused vials were still here in Amersfoort. I wanted to know whether it was possible to inject the 714X directly into the tumor and whether it was still safe to use the vials. I had understood from Saul that it was very important to get rid of the tumors, because the tumors were ticking time bombs. Cerbe replied that they recommended using 714X by injection only. It needed to be injected in the lymphatic system to work. I discussed the 714X therapy with Benjamin, and he said that this was the last treatment he was willing to try. Now I needed to solve the problem of where I would get the syringes from and who would be willing to help Benjamin administer the injections, as I knew he would never want to do it himself. He felt he needed medical assistance with the injections.

In the meantime I also tried to find out where I could order vitamin B-17 IVs. [51] Laetrile had been very helpful the first year Benjamin had been diagnosed with cancer. It had helped tremendously to reduce the tumor markers, without any side effects. The company I had ordered it from in the past had disappeared; their phone number was no longer in service, nor could I find them on the Internet. Was this another case where the FDA had raided them and made sure they would no longer operate their business? I finally found a company in Mexico that could supply the Laetrile. I placed an order and hoped that the vials would arrive soon.

In the meantime I was looking for answers: *How was it possible that the tumor markers were rising so quickly? Why was Benjamin's health deteriorating so rapidly? Why did he still have a large tumor in his neck?* These and the other questions I did not have answers to overwhelmed me. Looking back, I can see that we were in denial, but it was impossible for me to see that at the time. Just a year ago his tumor markers were all back to normal; tumors had been pushed out of his body, his testicle had been removed, yet his health was going downhill. Even though we knew that tumors remained after the testicle was removed, we wondered why they had not disappeared while he was receiving chemo treatment. The

---

51.   Vitamin B-17, also known as Laetrile or Amygdalin.

neck tumor had been biopsied twice, and I realized that we had never received a proper report from the doctors.

I decided to ask Dr. Hoekman for the biopsy report. I wanted to know; I needed answers, especially because Benjamin was experiencing a lot of backaches lately. He was not sleeping or eating well. He was becoming rather thin and only weighed 138 pounds. I was hoping that this was not because his tumor markers were increasing. I had so many unanswered questions.

Besides Dr. Hoekman, I also e-mailed Dr. Witjes, the specialist who had removed the testicle. I wanted to know whether he had already advised Dr. Schellart about the blood tests. I also wanted to know whether the tumors in Benjamin's abdomen had fluid. If so, would it be possible to have it drained, in the hope that would make Benjamin more comfortable?

My friend oncologist from the United States had told me that if the tumor was spongelike, with many small pockets of fluid, then drainage was not possible. He said that intraperitoneal therapy was pretty effective at diminishing the reaccumulation of fluid. That meant a needle would be inserted and as much fluid as possible evacuated. Then a solution of a chemotherapy drug would be injected; the patient is then rolled around to allow the chemo to make contact with as much of the tumor as possible. Since it is not injected intravenously there are essentially no side effects, and the medication goes exactly where it should go. I asked Dr. Witjes whether this was a possibility, as I knew Benjamin had made it absolutely clear to me that typical chemotherapy was not an option. I don't think I ever received an answer to that question. I am not even sure whether that type of therapy was even being used here in the Netherlands.

At the time of all this stress and worrying about Benjamin and trying to find out the status of his disease, we had a wedding coming up. Benjamin's cousin Jason was getting married on February 2 in the United States, and our relatives in the States were still waiting for an answer whether we were going to attend. We had received an official invitation by then, and I needed to respond and return the card. I still had not made up my mind. In the back of my mind I was hoping that Benjamin's disease was not as bad as I was afraid of and that we would all still be able to travel to New Jersey. It was important that Benjamin first had a blood test to find out whether his tumor markers had risen. If so we knew for sure that the cancer was active again. The result would help clarify the decision of whether to cross the Atlantic or not.

Besides the wedding, we also had our move to a much larger house to consider. We were planning to move before March 1. The new place was perfect for Benjamin. It meant he finally would have space to invite and entertain his friends. Yet I would be close by in case he needed assistance or someone to look after him. He was already planning the layout and looking at different ways of furnishing and decorating his new home.

A few days after I e-mailed Dr. Witjes, I received a reply from him. He was certain, without a doubt, that the cancer in Benjamin's abdomen was once again active. He told me that the pain was probably caused not by the tumor mass but by ingrowth, which meant that the tumor wasn't growing against but into another structure. He mentioned that intraperitonial chemo was not without side effects and that we would not reach the tumor in Benjamin's case. In other words, he did not think it was an option. There was no doubt in his mind that the tumors makers would have risen tremendously.

I wanted to know from him what therapy he suggested or whether it was valuable to start another therapy at all. I wanted to know whether chemotherapy was ever successful. After reading the book *Questioning Chemotherapy* by Ralph Moss, PhD[52] and the heartbreaking story about Alexander[53], a little boy that died of cancer, I did have doubts about chemotherapy. In Benjamin's case the tumor was growing into his spine. The only available option was very intensive chemotherapy and an operation afterward. Last September an operation had been impossible because of the enormous tumor mass and the risks of the operation. The operation would only be possible if chemotherapy reduced the tumor mass enormously. Dr. Witjes did not expect that result because the first rounds of chemotherapy had not reduced the mass. The chances that secondary chemotherapy would do so were definitely less than the primary treatment, and therefore the future did not look bright.

52.   Ralph W. Moss, PhD, *Questioning Chemotherapy* (Brooklyn, NY: Equinox Press, 1995).
53.   See http://www.ouralexander.org

I began to get extremely worried about Benjamin, especially after Dr. Witjes' information. It was like déjà vu all over again. It was time again to connect with my medical friends outside of Holland. I started digging into the Internet, looking for answers once more, trying to discover if there were any new developments on cancer in general. I found information on C-Statin, an herbal angiogenesis inhibitor.[54] I read about natural angiogenesis inhibitors named Angiostatin and a second natural inhibitor, Endostatin. I wrote to Dr. Schachter, letting him know that Benjamin was suffering backaches and that we were afraid the cancer was active again. I informed him that Benjamin had finally had his testicle removed, but that a large tumor mass remained in his abdomen; there were tumors near his lungs and a large visible tumor mass in his neck. I told him that the chemotherapy had done nothing to reduce the tumor mass. I wanted to know what his findings were with Poly-MVA and CAAT therapies[55] and whether he would recommend any of these therapies for Benjamin.

I also let him know that I had found a young alternative doctor here in the Netherlands who sounded promising. This young doctor had actually spoken personally with Dr. Schachter when he had been to Dr. Schachter's ACAM lectures in the United States. I had asked this young doctor whether he was willing to follow Dr. Schachter's protocol and wondered whether Dr. Schachter was willing to forward him the medical plan. I believed in Dr. Schachter's protocol, and to this day I am convinced that if Benjamin had not been so difficult and stubborn in the beginning and had followed his suggestion to have the testis removed right away and then followed through with the protocols Dr. Schachter had suggested, he would have been cured. The Laetrile had definitely been effective in reducing Benjamin's tumor markers.

As always, Dr. Schachter responded to my e-mail immediately. He did not recommend CAAT at this time but felt that Poly-MVA

54.　　An old American Indian remedy.

55.　　Poly-MVA is a nontoxic, powerful antioxidant formula. Dr. Merrill Garnett, a doctor and research chemist, is the inventor of Poly-MVA. He saw cancer as the failure of cells to regenerate normally. Poly-MVA restores healthy pathways for growth and normal development within the cell, and controls the cancer, rather than "fight[s] the cancer" and poison the system. See http://en.wikipedia.org/wiki/Merrill_Garnett; www.polymva.org/polymva_products-inventor.htm. CAAT is Controlled Amino Acid Treatment. See www.mbschachter.com/articles_&_literature.htm and www.apjohncancerinstitute.org/.

was a reasonable option, although very expensive. He did know about the C-Statin. The herb is a bindweed, also known as vascustatin. He recommended three bindweed products, which Benjamin could use along with vitamin C drips. He also pointed out a new, relatively inexpensive protocol[56] involving certain nutrients, some in very high doses. There had been many testimonials with objective evidence of cancer reversal in even very advanced cases. He suggested setting up a phone consultation between him, Benjamin, and me.

Ten days had passed since we first heard that our family physician was uncomfortable issuing a referral for the blood test. Ten valuable days were wasted; ten days spent not knowing what was going on in Benjamin's body, ten days when doctors did nothing to speed the process of discovery. All we needed was a simple referral from our family doctor to request that Benjamin's Alfa Foeto Protein, beta HCG, and LDH levels be checked. I asked Witjes if he could send a referral to the Lichtenberg Hospital in Amersfoort and leave Dr. Schellart out of the picture altogether so that we could take care of the blood work the next day. Witjes was beginning to get annoyed with me. He felt things were beginning to get complicated. How differently Dutch doctors reacted toward their clients compared to their colleagues in the United States … I had experienced nothing but very helpful doctors and specialists in the United States, regardless of whether I was a client or not. Whenever we contacted specialists in the United States, they were always more than helpful. They would even take the time to call me personally on the phone. What was the problem here in Holland? Didn't they see the urgency?

I e-mailed Dr. Schellart and once again asked for a referral, detailing exactly what factors needed to be identified in the referral. I wondered who was the doctor here? What was so difficult? What was he afraid of? I also assured him that he would not need to do the analyses; those would be done in either Nijmegen or Amsterdam. All he needed to do was to write up this referral for the local hospital in Amersfoort to save us from traveling a couple of hours to the other hospitals. Benjamin was now experiencing such an intense backache that it was not comfortable at all for him to sit in a car for over an hour or two. I told our family

---

56.   www.ncrf.org

doctor that I would be picking up the referral the next morning. At long last, on January 14, Benjamin went to our local hospital to have the blood test done.

All this arranging and following up on everything and everyone was getting to me. It all needed to be done early in the morning or in the evening, because I was still working full time as a freelance consultant in The Hague. I felt I needed to take a few days away from work, or to perhaps work from home, because not working meant no income. I then found out that in the Netherlands you can apply for a short sick leave, up ten days per year, to take care of your children, relatives, or family and that the employer will still pay 70 percent of your salary. It would give me time to take Benjamin to the hospital for tests; it would give me time to do further research and to nurse Benjamin.

It was almost the middle of January. His health was deteriorating rapidly. I noticed that he was extremely tired; he stayed in bed a lot of the time, and he was barely eating. He was experiencing a lot of pain. He had difficulties sleeping; during the night I could hear him scream from the pain. However, during the day he never complained or let me know that there was anything wrong.

For some reason Benjamin felt he had to "protect" me, and therefore he did not discuss how he was really feeling. But I could read the pain in his eyes; I could see it in his face. Walking was becoming difficult, and he grew thinner by the day. These were all signs that the cancer was very active, I knew. We did not really need a blood test to come to that conclusion. My heart ached for Benjamin. I wished I could take his pain away, wished he could be a happy and healthy twenty-four-year-old.

I talked to Benjamin what needed to be done, and he was all for trying the 714X, but he said that was the final effort he was going to make. He did not want further therapies and definitely not conventional therapies. He was also willing to start the Laetrile IVs again, if we could find a doctor or clinic that was willing and capable of administering them.

The young doctor who knew Dr Schachter was a potential option. The problem was that he was a long car ride away. We needed to find someone closer. It all seemed much more of an effort than it had been in the United States. I had already ordered the Laetrile in Mexico and was waiting for it to arrive. In the meantime I followed up with Dr. Hoekman, the oncologist in Amsterdam who I had asked in the beginning of the month about the results of the second neck tumor biopsy. He finally responded by asking for my correct address so that he could send the results. To this day I am still waiting for these results. He informed me that no malignant cells had been found in the neck tumor. He said this was not proof that the tumor was not cancerous, because he claimed the chemo had probably killed all the malignant cells. I did not understand. That tumor had been biopsied twice; both times the tumor mass had been found benign. The first time it was biopsied in the United States, Benjamin had not yet received chemotherapy, so Dr. Hoekman's conclusion did not make sense at all. Why couldn't they answer my question about what this neck tumor was? If they did not know, and obviously they didn't, what was I to think of the conventional medical world? Yet they were very quick to condemn all alternative therapies and to call the medical professionals who did work with nonconventional treatments "quacks." Dr. Hoekman asked how Benjamin was doing, as he claimed Benjamin had a special place in his heart. I responded that Benjamin was not doing well and that he was experiencing terrible pain. I asked what could be done against the pain.

At the same time I also contacted a professor in the University Medical Center (UMC), Utrecht, about an article I had read in the paper. This article was very optimistic about results with angiostatins; I understood from the article that the UMC was going to extend their tests with a few more patients. I was wondering whether they would consider Benjamin.

I also asked Dr. Hoekman about anti-angiogenic therapy because I did not think chemotherapy was any longer an option for Benjamin. Both Benjamin and I no longer believed in chemotherapy, especially after reading that "chemotherapy is basically ineffective in the vast majority of cases in which it is given."[57] I asked Dr. Hoekman what new developments were going on in the VU (University Hospital in Amsterdam) and what alternatives they could provide. He could not offer any options. Instead he let me know that he agreed with Dr. Moss that chemo did not really work and that Benjamin's tumors were not

---

57.   Ralph Moss, *Questioning Chemotherapy*, page 81.

operable, nor would radiation do any good. He confirmed that a lot of attention was being paid to antiangiogenic therapy, but that was all.

For the pain, he suggested Vioxx 25 mg or Thalidomide 200 mg per day. Vioxx was later in the news and was withdrawn from the U.S. market in 2004 due to concerns about an increased risk of heart attacks and stroke. A side effect of taking Vioxx, I now know, was abdominal pain. Vioxx had first been prescribed to Benjamin as a painkiller when he was still living in the United States. I now wonder whether this drug was one of the reasons he always felt so bad and why he experienced abdominal pain. It seems the conventional medical world at times is at a loss and does not always know what they are doing. Other questions I asked about different techniques and therapies, like laser techniques, were never answered.

From Dr. Schachter I received a full explanation of the Eichorn protocol.[58] I had looked the protocol up on the Web, and it all looked very promising. It made sense to schedule a telephone consultation for Benjamin and I with Dr. Schachter to discuss this protocol and other potential options. The call was scheduled for January 28. I also contacted Eichorn myself and explained our present situation, explaining that Benjamin was no longer following any conventional therapy and that he was not on any medication, either for his pain or for the cancer. I explained that we were considering the nontoxic therapy 714X, which supports the lymphatic and immune systems. I had finally found a local orthomolecular doctor who was willing to help to inject the 714X. Together with this therapy we wanted to follow Mr. Eichorn's vitamin program.

Our first appointment with the orthomolecular doctor was scheduled for January 17. The first meeting was to get to know each other and to discuss exactly what protocol we were going to follow. We would also discuss the Eichorn vitamin program.

I was also looking for therapies that could reduce the tumor mass. My friend Saul had told me that we needed to get rid of the tumors, which were ticking time bombs. Once cancer came back, it was far more difficult to treat. Again I contacted Dr. Witjes. I wanted a report

---

58.   The Eichorn protocol was developed by Fred Eichorn, It is a vitamin and mineral supplementation protocol. For more details please visit www.ncrf.org/

on Benjamin's abdominal tumors; I wanted to know what the tumors were. Nobody had been able to tell me in the past years exactly what those tumors were. I also wanted him to forward all the medical reports to Dr. Felperlaan, the orthomolecular doctor. Dr. Witjes was not willing to help. He did not want to mail reports about his patient. Our family doctor should supply us with records. Well, the family doctor was not of much use either. He had been my doctor for almost thirty years, but when I really needed him he was not there for us. He explained that because his practice was in Bunschoten he could not come down to Amersfoort. All this unwillingness and e-mailing back and forth was costing valuable time. I began to feel that we were running out of time, and I was getting desperate. Benjamin was not doing well at all. He now was in pain twenty-four hours a day; all he did was lie on his bed or on the couch in the living room.

Urgently, out of hopelessness, I contacted Dr. Hoekman to tell him that the painkillers did not work. I wrote that as I mother, I had to watch powerlessly as my son became sicker by the day; he was losing weight and, worst of all, he was in agony every day and had been for weeks now. I needed Dr. Hoekman to prescribe a strong drug against the pain. I asked him to fax the prescription to our local pharmacy. Dr. Hoekman wrote that if the painkillers did not work, the only option was morphine medication. He felt it was time for Benjamin to come to the hospital as an outpatient and suggested a mild form of chemotherapy and morphine. He obviously did not "get" the message and did not realize how serious the situation was becoming.

On January 17, we visited Dr. Felperlaan in Baarn. I immediately liked him, and so did Benjamin. He was a gentle man, full of understanding, and very willing to help Benjamin. I had brought Eichorn's vitamin protocol, the 714X vials, and the syringes I had ordered online. I also had specific instructions for how to administer the 714X, which must be introduced directly into the lymphatic system. We would visit Dr. Felperlaan for the daily injection for a total of twenty-one days starting on Monday, January 21.

I was pleased with the visit, and I became hopeful again. Benjamin wanted to do the 714X therapy together with the vitamin C and Laetrile IVs. Optimistic, I mentioned a Dutch saying to Benjamin: "Drie maal is scheepsrecht," which means three times lucky. I meant that this time

Benjamin might really beat his cancer and become a healthy young man. He, however, he interpreted it the other way round, that the third time might mean the end. He began to give me all sorts of hints, trying to let me know in a careful way that the end might be near. He would make comments like, "All I want to do is die in dignity. I will not make the end of the month. I am sorry I will not be able to see Sarah grow up." Through little statements like these, he was telling me that this time he would not recover.

On Monday January 21, Benjamin did not visit Dr. Felperlaan. Benjamin had started using morphine patches, which were making him even sicker. Down in the garage on our way to the car to visit the doctor, he had to throw up; he felt awful. He could barely stand on his feet. I took him back upstairs to the apartment and told him to lie down and stay home. We would try again the next day. Dr. Felperlaan had read the protocol in detail and had everything prepared and ready when we arrived the next day. Everything went as planned, and Benjamin received the 714X injection without any problem. However, the second day when we visited Dr. Felperlaan it did not work. Benjamin was lying on the examination table, ready to receive his injection. When the needle entered the injection site in the groin area, Benjamin screamed, his screams filled with pain. Benjamin burst out crying. He could not stand the pain, and Benjamin was not afraid of needles at all. The doctor withdrew the needle and we stopped treatment.

God only knows how many needles had been stuck into Benjamin to draw blood over and over again. Seeing him in so much pain was unbearable. I could barely stand it. What you go through you when your child is in such pain is indescribable. I needed to leave the room. I was dizzy. My heart ached for Benjamin. Tears came to my eyes. Perhaps that was the only time I asked "Why?": a question with no answer, a useless question. But at such a time a mother is so very helpless, unable to help. I could only stand there and watch my son suffer. How long did this suffering need to go on? Had he not suffered enough? *Why, for God's sake, why? What was the purpose of all this?*

On January 22 we at last received the result from the blood test. The news was not good, not good at all. The beta HCG was still in order. The LDH (lactate dehydrogenase) and AFP levels had risen considerably and had increased more than tenfold. The numbers were not as bad as back in May 2000, but it was obvious that the cancer was very active. I passed the test results on to Al, my United States oncologist friend, because I wanted his opinion. I also wanted to know whether he was aware of testicular cancer cases where the tumor mass had not shrunk, as in Benjamin's case. Neither the chemotherapy nor the Laetrile therapy had done anything to reduce the tumor mass, but both therapies had been successful in reducing the tumor makers dramatically. That was something I did not understand. According to Al, it was quite common for one component of a mixed testicular tumor to respond to chemotherapy but not another. I also contacted Saul and Mark, my alternative medical friends, because I was now more than just worried. Something had to be done quickly. Benjamin was not eating and was losing weight, and I needed to know whether the hydrazine sulphate I had was still good and what dosage I should start him on. I also needed to know if there were any food restrictions—not that it mattered a great deal, because Benjamin was not eating anyway, which was why I wanted to start him on the hydrazine sulphate, a medication that stimulated the appetite. It blocks the action of a liver enzyme called PEP-CK, which the liver uses to convert lactic acid (cancer's waste) to glycogen (sugar). When this enzyme is blocked by hydrazine sulphate, the cancer is deprived of its endless supply of sugar. Then it calls for more sugar, and appetite returns. Saul as always responded immediately.

In addition to answering my questions, he made me aware of a new therapy called IPT: Insulin Potentiation Therapy. The doctor injects insulin, which drives sugar out of the blood. The cancer cells, which use twenty times more sugar than regular cells, open up to get all the sugar they can. After an hour, a tiny bit of chemo is injected. At that time, when the cancer cells are wide open, they take in the chemo and die. IPT therapy destroys the tumor mass. This therapy had apparently worked for some people for whom ozone could not complete the job. After IPT, ozone could then clean up the toxins in the system. Benjamin had not been in his ozone steam sauna since the testicle had been removed in June. He had been so convinced that he had beaten the cancer that he thought the daily saunas were no longer necessary.

I decided to search the Internet for IPT therapy, as it sounded very promising. IPT was available from twenty-six doctors worldwide in five countries, including the United States, Canada, Mexico, Argentina, and Ecuador. The first European doctors would be trained in IPT in early 2002. I was determined to find a doctor who could provide this therapy. Through the IPT Web site, I contacted Mr. Chris Duffield, PhD, who was very helpful and informed me that I was in luck; Dr. Jean Remy Lepan in France had just received IPT training from Dr. Perez Garcia the previous week. He would return from the United States the following week. Unfortunately there were no trained doctors yet in the Netherlands. I e-mailed Dr. Lepan to let him know we were desperately seeking answers and that I was wondering whether IPT therapy was a possibility. I asked him to let me know where he was located and what exactly the treatment included.

In the meantime, Benjamin tried to start the ozone therapy again, but he was very uncomfortable and could not sit for long because of severe back pain. He had stopped the morphine patches because they made him throw up several times a day. Without the patches he felt not as sick, but he was in pain again all day long. He tried to reduce the pain by smoking marijuana, but Benjamin did not really want to do that because it made him high. Apparently there was some kind of device you could use that gave you the pain reducing benefits without making you high. We bought the device, called a vaporizor. It is used for heating dried plants and herbs without burning them, allowing you to inhale the therapeutic oils of the plants. In the end Benjamin never used the device because it shouldn't be used on an empty stomach. And Benjamin was not eating. To get him to eat, I started Benjamin on the hydrazine sulfate. January 24 was the first day Benjamin took the medication. He started with one tablet in the morning. If what I had read about the product was true, Benjamin's appetite should have returned in a couple of days, and he'd want to eat again. He needed to get some food in him; he needed to regain some strength. I also bought all the vitamins that Fred Eichorn had recommended. According to the protocol, Benjamin had to take more than fifty tablets a day. I was worried about the large number because Benjamin had great difficulties swallowing so many pills; plus he should not take them on an empty stomach. Eichorn's assistant was very helpful and suggested we grind up the pills and make a shake by adding milk, yogurt, or fruit drinks, anything that he liked that would make the blend tasty.

The Laetrile still had not arrived; it seemed to take forever. Therefore the chances that we could start the Laetrile protocol at all became very slim. I was disturbed that Laetrile was no longer for sale in the United States. The company in Rochester where I used to order the Laetrile was no longer there. The FDA had published some bad articles over the past year, and CNN amongst others reported on it. I thought it was disgusting that people could not choose their own therapies. Chemo does not always cure, but while it was okay to use poison, the FDA had banned a harmless apricot seed. How crazy was that?

We had stopped the 714X therapy, not just because it had been a very painful experience but also because Benjamin was becoming more bedridden. He barely got out of bed now and was wasting away. His health had deteriorated even more.

I still tried to work as a consultant as much as I could. I worked from home for several days because I needed to earn an income. I asked Wayne to come by and visit with Benjamin every day, not only to support Benjamin as much as he could but also to help with small things, such as getting medication from the pharmacy and other such tasks. We also needed to find a new family doctor who would be willing to make house visits. To make Benjamin more comfortable and to include him more in our day-to-day living and to avoid isolating him in his small bedroom, we placed a single bed in the living room, just under the front window, facing the TV. I bought a large TV and DVD player; since our return from the United States we had been watching TV on a very small twenty-eight-inch screen. I hoped that the new TV and DVD player would help Benjamin feel a bit better and distract him from his pain. Benjamin was now back on morphine patches to help him cope with the pain.

As word spread that Benjamin was not doing well, I began to receive more e-mails from relatives and friends. Kathleen, Benjamin's friend from Austin, who had visited him a year ago during the Christmas holidays had been trying unsuccessfully to call, and she now e-mailed me. She was very concerned for him. She had heard from Zoë that he was not eating and that he was not getting out of bed. She wished she could come and help take some of the burden off of me. She asked me to get back to her and give her a more definitive description of his status. It really meant a lot to her, and she had many questions.

I began to realize it was time I contacted my friends and relatives overseas to update them. They were always anxious to hear the latest developments. I informed them that Benjamin was back on morphine so that he could get a bit of rest. His rapid decline was quite unbelievable. Only four weeks before he had played music at Zoë's birthday party; twenty-eight days later he lost tons of weight and could not do anything anymore. I told them that Benjamin and I had talked about death a couple of times over the past couple of days, and that all he wanted from me was to let him die with dignity when the time came. He did not want to go back into a hospital; he did not want any more chemo. He made me promise that no matter what happened I would take care of him at home.

Benjamin and I talked about the fact that his stay in the hospital had been his worst nightmare. Never again did he want to go through that experience. It took me back to the time my father was dying, and we, his immediate family, against his will had taken him back to the hospital. And he had used the last bit of his strength to tell us to please get him out. We did so, and a day later he had died peacefully in his own home. The thought that my son was dying was heartbreaking, but I was not yet ready to accept it. In my eyes we still had lots of alternatives, different therapies we could try. I was in denial, although in the back of my mind I knew we were running out of time. I felt that if I could replenish his strength, if he would begin to eat again, we could gain some time, and perhaps a miracle would happen. I desperately researched all sorts of alternatives and hoped we weren't too late.

Benjamin, however, believed that he was dying and that he would not get well again. He seemed to be at peace with the idea that this might be it. He was not much interested in any alternative therapies anymore, or any therapy, for that matter. I think he just took the medication and pills to comfort me, not so much for his own sake.

On the last day of January I received an e-mail from Dr. Lepan in France. His English was rather broken, and some of his sentences were not clear to me. But the conclusion of the e-mail was that Benjamin would need to come to France for the therapy twice a week for the first two weeks and then once a week, for a total of six weeks. Sadly, Benjamin by then was in no condition to travel anywhere; he was almost 100 percent bedridden. He got up from his bed only to go to the bathroom, and he was able to manage that only with help from me. The previous night I had spoken to Dr. Schachter. Benjamin had not taken part in the phone conversation, as he was not feeling up to it. Dr. Schachter did not have much good news either, apart from the vitamin therapy he had recommended. He did tell me that he had good experiences with the hydrazine sulfate Benjamin was now taking for his appetite. I was hoping that the hydrazine sulfate would work soon and that Benjamin would start eating; once he was strong enough, I could take him to Dr. Lepan in France. Once he started the hydrazine sulfate, I began to keep a daily journal. After he had been on the hydrazine sulfate for five days, Benjamin still showed no desire to eat. As a matter of fact, some mornings he was so much in pain that he did not even drink the orange-carrot juice I made for him first thing each morning.

On February 1 I received an e-mail from Dr. Hoekman, in response to my e-mail from ten days earlier. He said he could tell that the situation was getting worse and unfortunately he could not do much. He wondered whether it would still be useful to give Benjamin a mild form of chemo as an outpatient. But he doubted whether this would do him any good. In case of unacceptable pain, he suggested increasing the Durogesic in small increments. He closed by saying to contact him again when the situation at home became intolerable.

Wayne now visited every day, and I had stopped my consultancy work altogether for the time being. Benjamin was very down; he said he would die before the end of the month. How could he know that? I would not believe it, I did not want to believe it—I was not giving up. He still looked reasonably good in my eyes, much better than when he was in the hospital. His tumor markers weren't as bad as they had been when he was admitted to the VU hospital in May 2000. I was not just going to surrender. I was going to make sure we would win this battle. I still had a lot of hope for Benjamin.

But did Benjamin have hope? It was obvious he was getting sicker by the day. He could not get out of bed at all. I now had to help him with everything: to bathe him, brush his hair, make him comfortable by turning him. Changing the bed was a challenge because he could not sit up, and I had to take the sheets off bit by bit and replace them with clean ones while I gently turned him from his left to his right side, but somehow I managed. I cried most of the day. Tears ran down my face, and I couldn't stop them. I did try not to for Benjamin's sake. But how could I not cry when my child was so totally dependent, in so much pain, dying right in front of me? Benjamin said he wished he could cry along with me, but he could not. The only time he cried during those few days before he died was when he watched the music video *Prince in Concert: Rave Un2 the Year 2000* by his greatest hero, Prince.

Benjamin's birthday was on February 2. My son, beautiful on both the outside and inside, was now twenty-four years old. How different his birthday was compared to last year's surprise party for him. Last year he was doing so well. He had made a remarkable recovery, we thought. He had put on a lot of weight and enjoyed life. He went out with his friends, was very much into his music, recorded it on his computer; he experimented with different Web sites, wondering how he could share his cancer experience and what he could do to better the world. He was so full of hope then. And now, just twelve months later, he was totally bedridden, losing weight, not eating and in pain twenty-four hours a day.

Family and friends dropped by during the day. February 2 was a Saturday, and people were off work. Although it was nice of them to drop by, it was too much for Benjamin. He was very, very tired and having to listen to all those people talk was too much for him.

His birthday came and went. I don't think Benjamin had really enjoyed it. Again he had not eaten. He still hadn't responded to the hydrazine sulfate pills. I had read everything there was to read about it; for some people it had worked miracles pretty quickly, but most saw results within two or three weeks. I still hoped that the hydrazine sulfate would start working and that it was not too late. Benjamin took three tablets a day and had been taking them for eight days, and even though he was still not eating, he said he wanted to. Then later one day he asked for a small piece of birthday cake and actually ate a couple of very small pieces. I was delighted and hopeful. Finally he was getting something solid into him, even if it was only cake. I was still hoping that once the hydrazine sulfate began to work, he would be able to regain his energy and we could consider going to France for the IPT therapy.

On February 5 Benjamin was pretty down again, and again he told me he did not think it would take very long before the end came. He said he could feel tumors all through his body. And still I would not hear of it.

I continued with my research and contacted my doctor friends for answers, but none of them had any answers or suggestions anymore. I think they already realized that Benjamin was not going to make it; only I was hanging on to the last straw.

Mike was becoming worried about me and spoke about having Benjamin admitted into the hospital or hospice. That was something I definitely did not want to hear. "No," I said. "No, no, no. I will not have him admitted; I promised Benjamin I would take care of him myself, no matter what."

"But," Mike argued, "what if it becomes too much, too heavy, for you?"

I did not care; I would look after him no matter what. By then I was sleeping on the couch in the living room so that I was nearby during the night. Benjamin had not slept through the night for a long time; he was worried that if he needed my help I would not hear him if I slept in my bedroom.

On Wednesday, February 6, Benjamin seemed to feel a bit better. Our new family doctor came by to visit. He was a young doctor from Belgium who was temporarily helping out in a doctors' practice just down the road from where we lived. His name was Dr. Tom van den Eede. Benjamin liked him right away. Benjamin told him that he did not want to be admitted to a hospital, that he definitely did not want any more chemotherapy, and that he just wanted to die in dignity at home. Dr. van den Eede respected his wishes and seemed very understanding. Benjamin also requested new morphine patches for the pain. Dr. van den Eede wrote out the prescription and promised before he left that he would drop by every other day or so.

During the day Benjamin asked for some food; he wanted a slice of Dutch *ontbijtkoek*[59] and a cookie. He also ate a peanut butter sandwich. He even asked for potato chips and some nuts! It seemed that the

---

59.   Breakfast cake

hydrazine sulfate was beginning to work. During the day and evening we had several visitors. My mother, who was recovering from a knee operation, dropped by, along with my brother and sister-in-law. Later Arjan, Benjamin's cousin, Zoë, Frido, Wayne, and Emmelien and her mother visited. Emmelien was the girl Benjamin had fallen in love with just half a year before, when he was still very mobile and did not realize that the cancer was active again, back when he still went out in the evenings with his friends.

Emmelien's mother was a breast cancer survivor, and Benjamin had wanted to talk to her. They had never met but they got on well. Benjamin talked a lot with Emmelien and her mother. They had fun; Benjamin actually laughed several times. It was good to see him enjoying some moments during these depressing days. The following night he again did not sleep. He drank some orange and carrot juice and ate a slice of bread, half an apple, and half an orange. In the morning I changed the bed, and Benjamin mentioned that he would like to read his e-mails. Since he had moved to the bed in the living room and become bedridden, he had not touched his computer. Mike and I thought perhaps if we could sit him up, with lots of pillows behind his back, we could place his computer on a side table so he could access his e-mails. That was a big mistake. Benjamin was too weak; we could not get him in an upright position. And it was too painful. It was heartbreaking to see my son so defenseless, so vulnerable, and unable to even sit up somewhat. The hurt I experienced is indescribable.

I called the local medical supplier for a hospital bed that could be raised automatically so that Benjamin could sit up somewhat, plus a hospital table that would fit over his bed. That way we could place his computer in front of him so he could check his mails. The bed and table were going to be delivered the following Tuesday, early in the morning.

While he was bedridden, I tried to be as close as I could to Benjamin. I tried to make him as comfortable as possible. I caressed him softly wherever it was not painful, where no tumors protruded from his body, and massaged his feet. In the evening he had two bites of pasta and asked for chips again. During the days, we spoke a lot about the past. Benjamin wanted to talk about when he was small, about the fun things we did, about his school years. He also reminisced about his friends, his cousins, and all of those who had been important in his life. He said how sorry he was that he would not be able to see his little sister Sarah grow up. We talked about my parents, what a kind and gentle character my mother was, how fond he had been of my father. We talked about what he wanted me to do with his things after he passed, who was going to get what. He wanted me to have his papers. His papers? I did not understand until after Benjamin died and I found his story. We talked about where he wanted to be buried, whether he wanted an official service—all the details I did not want to discuss but that needed to be discussed.

Benjamin did not find it hard to discuss these matters. It seemed he had made peace with it all, and he taking care of the last bits and loose ends. He asked Mike to sit down with him, and he discussed their relationship, which had not always been without problems; he said he held no hard feeling toward Mike.

I told him that even though I knew he was not really interested in taking all the pills, vitamins, and medications I put in front of him anymore, I felt that I needed to do so, because if I did not keep trying until the end I would feel guilty after he passed about not having done enough. I would not be able to live with myself if I had not done everything that I could, including simply putting out all his pills, even if he refused to take them. Benjamin assured me that I was strong enough and that I would be okay. He was not very worried about me; he was sure that I would be able to cope and carry on with life once he had stepped out of his.

He asked Klaas to come over that Sunday. He wanted to spend some quality time alone with him, his best friend, his buddy, with whom he had shared the good and the bad since they were little kids of barely three or four years old.

On Saturday, February 9, I had to attend the funeral for my ninety-five-year-old aunt. My mother had informed the priest about Benjamin. During the ceremony he mentioned that the son of a family member was terribly ill, and he asked everyone to pray for Benjamin. I sat there and cried, not for my aunt but for Benjamin, not realizing that exactly a week later I would be attending another funeral and burying my own son.

The day my aunt was buried was a busy day. After I got home from the funeral we had several visitors. Later in the afternoon Benjamin's father visited with his daughter Sarah and Zoë and Frido. Benjamin was exhausted, ready to give up. He wanted us to accept that he was dying; he wanted us to be at peace with it. His father was frustrated and told him he needed to keep on fighting—he could not give up. I felt very sorry for Benjamin and told Wayne to let him be, that he could fight no longer and that we should not force our selfish wills on him. Zoë was frustrated as well and asked Benjamin why he did not just end his life himself and get it over with if he did not want to live anymore or to try anymore. Why didn't he step out right now? It was all very sad, so very sad indeed. It was obvious that we all had a hard time dealing with the situation. We all loved him so much, and we did not want to lose him. We could not or did not want to understand that he was actually dying.

Zoë didn't mean those harsh words. The next day I explained to Benjamin that she had not meant it, that she had been expressing her frustration over dealing with it all. After all, her brother was everything to her. She had always protected Benjamin, beginning when he was just a little boy. If anyone touched Benjamin, they'd have to deal with her. She loved him dearly and always had. They had been very close their entire lives. Now to watch her little brother die was more than she could handle.

Saturday night Benjamin slept reasonably well. About fifteen days had gone by since he started taking the hydrazine sulfate, and he had started eating a tiny bit. I was still hopeful that he would regain some strength. I did not want to believe that Benjamin would not make the end of the month, like he had told me. In the afternoon Klaas dropped by, and I left them alone in the living room. I decided to clean Benjamin's bedroom up a bit and get his computer ready to move to the living room for when the hospital bed arrived Tuesday. Benjamin and Klaas talked for hours. I don't know what was discussed; at the time I did not realize that Benjamin was actually saying good-bye to Klaas. Klaas left late that afternoon looking rather distressed.

Benjamin had not drunk a lot of liquid that day, but he complained that his bladder felt full. He had not been able to pee since the day before, which worried him very much. His belly looked swollen and tight. I did not like it and was very troubled. The situation did not improve. At eight thirty that evening I decided to call the family doctor. Because it was Sunday nobody was at the practice; instead I was redirected to the weekend emergency service. I spoke to a doctor and explained the situation. However, there was nothing he could do, and he recommended that Benjamin be admitted to the hospital if the situation did not improve. He did not want to bother to drop by. We had to wait until the next morning, when I could reach Dr. van den Eede. In the meantime his condition worsened. Benjamin now started to hiccup, and he was getting heartburn. I felt powerless, anxious, and nervous. How were we going to make it through the night?

At one o'clock in the morning Benjamin said he needed to throw up. I quickly jumped off the couch and got a plastic bucket. He gave up a liter of very dark, almost black, liquid. I had never seen anything like it and did not know what it was. I decided to save some for the doctor to analyze the following day. I was worried, worried sick, to say the least. Benjamin on the other hand felt much relieved once he had thrown up. I guess the swollen feeling and the pressure on his bladder and belly had gone.

The next day was a lousy day; it poured with rain, just like the previous days. Rain and nothing but rain, and there seemed no end in sight. Dr. van den Eede came by and spoke a bit with Benjamin; he examined him and looked at the brown liquid I had saved for him. He knew exactly what it was but did not comment on it much. Maybe not to worry us ...

In the afternoon Klaas' s parents dropped by with a small puppy they wanted to show Benjamin. It was a cute, fluffy little white thing, and Benjamin enjoyed the playful dog. He seemed pleased and felt much better than the previous day. In the early evening Zoë came to visit; and she made up with Benjamin after their earlier fallout. They were again loving brother and sister. Benjamin adored his sister and had been very grateful to her for taking such good care of him when he first returned to Holland. He had said several times to me that he would not have known what to do without Zoë. He had written her a note on a small piece of paper when he DJ-ed for her birthday just over a month before, saying how much she meant to him. Those words were the last words he would ever write to her.

The next morning, February 12 (the Chinese New Year started that day), I got up pretty early and then washed and took care of Benjamin before eight o'clock. I wanted to get all that out of the way before the hospital bed was delivered around nine o'clock. While I was washing Benjamin, he said how tired he was and that he did not have any energy left; he was exhausted. He said he could not go on anymore. Then I spoke the words he probably had wanted to hear much sooner than that Tuesday: "Benjamin, why don't you let yourself go? It's okay."

He was all cleaned up and lying in bed, waiting for the hospital bed to arrive. Mike was in the kitchen making coffee. Then Benjamin said: "I want it to be a bit quiet this morning. Why don't you just sit down at the dining table, have your coffee together with Mike, and take it easy?"

Mike and I sat at the table, it was quiet. All of a sudden I thought I heard something. Mike said, "I think Benjamin is calling you." I looked over and saw Benjamin staring at the ceiling. I walked up to him and sat down on his bed. I held his hand. "Mike!" I called in panic, "What is going on? Why is he staring like that?" Mike walked up to Benjamin and kissed him on his forehead. Benjamin turned his head and looked at us, and I told him I loved him. Then he stared at the ceiling again. A deep breath followed, and his soul left his body very rapidly, flew out of the window, straight up into the sky.

The sun was shining; it was a beautiful day, a beautiful day to go up to heaven. Benjamin had passed. My brave and beautiful son was dead.

Afterword

During the three years that Benjamin, or should I say I, battled his cancer, I never truly knew how he felt about the ordeal. Perhaps I did not know because I was so obsessed with finding a cure for him, so blind to his spirituality that I did not realize that Benjamin himself was at peace with it. The few short statements I have included here and there throughout this book are pieces of his writing that I found after he had passed. Not until he died did I begin to understand, through his story and his entries in his journal, why he did what he did and why he behaved the way he did. All the pieces of the puzzle finally fell into place.

I first started writing this book shortly after he died, but I never was able to finish it, mainly because I had not actually dealt with his death like I thought. It would take a few years of ups and downs, emotional breakdowns, and crying for hours while I talked about it to my therapist before I could finally make the commitment to finish it.

Benjamin was a very spiritual person and looked at life very differently than young men his age typically did. I learned from his writing and speaking to his friends that he had undergone out-of-body experiences since he was fifteen or sixteen years old. Benjamin had never discussed these with me. He looked at life differently, perhaps because he had an old soul, as a Native American had told him, and therefore had much more life experience than I did. Through his battle Benjamin had struggled with whether he wanted to live or to die. In the end he choose for the latter.

Benjamin left me his papers when he died. He wanted me to find his story; he wanted me to write this book and show people there is more between heaven and earth and that there are many more therapies out there than just chemotherapy and radiation to treat cancer. Of course I wished he had lived, but I now understand that it had to be this way. I am at peace with it. I truly believe that nothing in this life is an accident and that Benjamin's dying young was predestined. The first signs were already there when he was first born, when I experienced those feelings that he was slipping through my hands as I held him. No matter what we did, or what we should have done, it would have made no difference. Neither the conventional nor the alternative therapies could have saved him. Benjamin was, this time around, purposely on this earth for a shorter period than most of us. He had no problem with it; it was we, his family, who did.

Benjamin's story

This story was discovered one day after Benjamin's death among his personal papers, the papers he wanted me to have. Benjamin handwrote it when he was only twenty years old, before he was diagnosed with cancer six months later.

December 26, 1998

The Boy and His Death

He was only twenty-four when they met. Death stood there, facing him. What used to make up his surroundings had disappeared. The boy examined Death closely and noticed the kind expression on his face. The boy must have looked puzzled when Death asked him what he wished to have answered. "I don't know where to start," the boy said. "There is so much I wish to know." Death lifted up his right arm, and with the motion clouds of dust appeared out of the blackness. Next, stars started forming, and finally a cover of white clouds appeared on a bright blue background. The feeling of ecstasy that had entered the boy's awareness together with death, slowly left. Something was pulling him down.

"What you are feeling now you have come to know as gravity," Death mentioned. The boy looked downward and noticed he was moving in that direction. Just a moment before, all sense of direction had disappeared. "You will get used to it," Death said to the boy. "But this feeling is awful," the boy replied.

"You have lived with it for twenty-four years."

"That's only because I didn't know any better."

"No, you did know better: gravity has a tendency to make you forget certain things. And it does more than that."

The boy and Death stopped falling. They had come to what seemed to be earth, just as it had been when the two of them had left it moments earlier. "What are we doing here?" the boy asked.

"There are certain things you have questions about. We are here to get the answers. But before we do, you will need to know the rules around here. First of all the rules of mankind, second the rules of nature, and third the rules of heaven. Once you know these, you are ready to begin getting the answers you are looking for." Death explained the rules to him.

"Do you have any questions you wished to have answered?" Death asked.

"Yes," the boy answered. "Have we met before?"

"I understand you have learned something," Death replied. "You surely remember your twenty-four years on earth. What you have forgotten is the time before you started your life again."

"Gravity has a tendency to make you forget certain things," the boy said, to his own surprise. At that moment he remembered how just moments ago he had lived a lifetime of seemingly twenty-four years. "But those twenty-four years were definitely real," the boy said, confused. Gravity also tends to slow things down a [bit] [great bunch]*. Here those years happen in an instant, yet it takes many people eternities to break through that barrier of time that comes with life. This time the feeling of ecstasy stayed.

"What happens next?" the boy asked.

"That is entirely up to you," Death replied. "During your (last) life you have learned how to use imagination, creativity. The world that was outside of you never changed, it was created by someone else. It was created to help you and only you reach a point where you would make your breakthrough. You have learned to move and find your way in imagination. You have learned that it is not outside, but inside yourself where it happens. You too are now a creator. You will embrace everything you see, hear, taste, smell, sense from now on."

"You mean I can create worlds, universes, just by imagining them?"

"Exactly."

"But what about you? You are here, and you are not part of my imagination."

"Yes, I am a creation of your imagination. A necessary part, because it is easy to forget that it is all your imagination and that's when we get lost in it [trying to ...]*.

"I will be here as your teacher for as long as you need me. There will come a time when you will remember how you created me by imagining me, and this is when I will depart and a student will arrive, and you will take my place and be the teacher. But this will be a whole new beginning of a whole new ending."

(For the next few eternities have some fun ...)

*Benjamin's original self-edits
© 1998 Benjamin Hyman

Beginning

December 31, 1998

Suddenly he realized the past twenty-four years were merely a creation of his imagination, which took place in a fraction of a moment. Those years never existed! In fact the whole concept of time started to lose its meaning.

"At some point you will forget that it is all your imagination," Death had told him. Like magic, Death appeared before him.

"But those years on earth were real! How can reality and imagination be so similar?" the boy asked. "That's because they are the same. They only differ in meaning, which we add to them. I prefer to use imagination, since reality seems to make us believe there is some sort of security we need to hold on to. An illusion that has tricked the best of them."

The boy could see clearly what the illusion held. Hey, he had lived it for twenty-four illusionary years. Over and over again. "What about my mother, my sister? Were they real?" the boy asked Death.

"Real in the sense you all shared the same illusion. In the illusion of your mother, you are her son. In your sister's illusion, you play the part of brother. Collective dreaming, I like to call it." (We all wake up sooner or later.)

"But now that I have woken up from my dream, what happens to my part in the illusions and dreams of the people close to me? Will I still exist to them?"

"This is difficult to explain but easy to understand. To them you disappeared out of what they call their lives. Where you went, they don't have a clue. They don't know you simply 'woke up.' In your case you woke up during their lives. So you weren't responding to their illusion of you anymore. To them you are dead. Just like your grandfather was to you. You are not the first who woke up from their illusion, you know."

"But I always thought he died of old age."

"No, in your illusion he was just old when he did. And so was he in his. Part of the collective dreaming you were part of was/is a belief system, that people are born the way you knew, grow old, and then die. Without this belief most would plainly never snap out of their illusion. Most, however, wake up and immediately go back to either a different illusion or the same one they just woke up from. That's is why it is important to create the right image of 'death' during your 'lifetime,' or illusion. You see, when you create a belief system about the afterlife, you are setting up your next dream. Some will be the victim of their own imagination and will find themselves far worse off then they were in their previous dream. At least in their previous dream they would eventually wake up (or die). Many people have at one point created their own eternity waiting for them in their next illusion. This is an illusion very hard to get out of, even with the help of others. I call it doom. You see, heaven and hell are basically the same when they both last an eternity."

Poof! Death was gone.

The boy started to look back at his illusion. His birth, his years growing up to be a child, his school years, finally his last years before he died of cancer. He understood that it was all part of his own imagination, and he recognized the blessing of his illness. It had enabled him to wake up to a place where he was the creator, a place where time had no meaning at all. A place without boundaries and limitations. A place where one and zero were the same. A place where his body had no beginning and no end. A place so magnificently free of everything that it wasn't even there. He also realized that what kept people from waking up was fear. He had spent most of his own illusion (life) dealing with the matter. Some people spend all their lives hiding from fear, then all their afterlives. But it is necessary to experience fear before being able to experience bliss. Yes, that's what it was, pure bliss!

That moment the boy knew he had a choice, a choice so wonderful it could only come from his imagination. He had a choice to grow old. To go back to his illusion and do all the things he was afraid of doing before he had imagined his death. To live life!

Death appeared. "This is something few people have done, or even dared do. You are willing to continue your illusion (dream) where you left off and to risk never waking up the way you just did. A lot can change during your dream of growing old. Especially since you are entering a collective dream. You might adopt belief systems that won't allow you to experience what you are experiencing now. Worst of all you might start ignoring imagination entirely. That is a common thing while growing old, you know."

"But I could help other people who haven't been as fortunate as me to experience all this and reach a deeper understanding of life and death, fear and bliss, sickness and health. So, that when they too are ready to wake up, they will be able to feel this. And maybe they then too will start helping others do the same. Isn't that what it is all about? To all wake up from this collective dream and reach our higher self?"

Note: The following was written but crossed out.

You died when you were twenty-four years old. When you go back you will be twenty again. It will be the last day of the year 1998. It will be up to you during those four years to decide. You were twenty-four when you ~~died~~ woke up. When you re-enter the collective dream you will be twenty again, and you will not remember any of this except in the form of a story you will write when you are back. It is a follow-up on the story you wrote five days earlier. Believe in it, always. Write more when you feel like it, then publish it when you are ready to wake up.

End crossed out text.

"Your intention is pure, and I will help you. Remember though, at one point you will start believing in things like reality and time. You will forget it is all your imagination. When this happens read this story and imagine. I will be there when you need me. I will keep teaching you the things you need to know, and occasionally meet you in your dreams."

The boy tried to think of an ending to his story. No matter how hard he tried, the right words to end the story wouldn't appear. Suddenly he realized there was no ending to this story. This was only the beginning ...

© December 31, 1998 Benjamin Hyman.

Dedicated to my only friend
He who will be there for me in the end
He who will take my pain away
On my final day
He who I can always count on
Even after I am gone
Death ...

© December 1998 Benjamin Hyman

Addendum

Last Week I Was a Criminal
Benjamin Hyman, April 1999

Earlier that night I had engaged in some heavy conversation with my mother. Afterward, both of us had sat in my car, crying. Knowing she was only going to be in Austin for a week, I felt angry at her. I started driving home, and I noticed three cats lying on the road. I steered around them, as they did not move out of the way. *That's odd*, I thought. Later, when I was going north on Loop 1, I spotted flashing lights in the distance. I slowed down. A terrible wreck appeared to have happened. There were three fire trucks, three ambulances, and a horde of police cars.

When I got to my apartment I was feeling frustrated. I still hadn't said to my mother what I had wanted to say to her for months. I decided to get in my car and drive. Driving always had a good effect on me. In a way I feel free whenever I drive. Especially through the Hills on a clear night with my roof open. That night I drove and I drove.

On my way home, I saw a flashing red traffic light too late and drove through it without stopping. Less than a minute later I got pulled over by a police officer. Soon after I stopped my car, my face was in the spotlight of the police man's bright flashlight. "Do you know why I stopped you?" he asked.

"Because I did not stop at the red flashing light?" I replied.

"You were speeding. Doing seventy miles an hour in a forty-five zone."

That's strange, I thought. I hadn't been speeding since I left my apartment. He asked me for my license and proof of insurance. I gave him what he asked for.

After I had been waiting in my car for five, maybe ten, minutes, the officer came back. He asked me to get out of the car, and before I knew it I was sitting in the back of a police car, handcuffed. He explained to me that I had an outstanding traffic ticket and that there was a warrant out for my arrest. The backup that had arrived, helped him search my car. They pulled a butterfly knife out of the back of my car. It was my butterfly knife. I had bought it in Greece, about four and a half years ago. I had forgotten all about that knife. *This must not look good*, I thought.

One of the two officers came back to the police car and asked me about the knife. I told him that it was mine.

During the ride to the West Lake police station, the police man told me that it was an illegal knife and that I could be charged with a class A misdemeanor. Possession of a prohibited weapon was a serious deal. Still handcuffed, I arrived at the station, where the officer told me to go through the glass door. I pointed toward the only door made of glass and said: "That door?" "No, that one," he said, while pointing at another door. *That's not a glass door*, I thought. It was a steel door with a thick plate of glass for a window next to it. I went in and started to think of all that had happened that night. I sat down with my hands still bonded behind my back. I wondered how long it would be before I would be out of there. Would I be out before the morning? It was the week before the last week in school, and I had to turn in my English assignment the next day. After an hour or so I got impatient. Weren't they supposed to be doing paperwork or something, so I could be transferred to the Austin Police Department? I overheard the two officers talking outside my cell. They weren't doing paperwork at all. Instead they were jokingly talking about some of the things that happened to them on the job. In their conversation I heard them use words like *motherfucker, shit, dick,* and *holy shit,* and I thought that it was not right for them to use such language, as these are the very people who are supposed to set the example for the rest of society. I heard one tell the other how this guy he had arrested earlier didn't deserve to see the daylight for the next five years. The situation started seeming worse than it had before. Not only had I gotten arrested, the people I had gotten arrested by seemed to have no moral values whatsoever. I couldn't wait to get to the headquarters in Austin, where I was sure the police would be of a better breed than the two I was at the mercy of now.

My mouth started to get dry. I needed a cup of water. I knocked on the glass. They ignored me. I knocked again. They still ignored me. I knocked again. After knocking four times, hoping one of the two would acknowledge me, I realized that these people didn't care about me. I sat back down, pulled my arms under my legs, placed my hand in front of me, and reached for my cigarettes and lighter. A few minutes later, one of the officers came to my cell. He opened the door and had an angry look on his face. He was not at all pleased that I was smoking and told me that he was going to cite me for violating city smoking laws. He also placed the cuffs back behind my back and told me if I didn't leave them behind my back he would tie me to the metal chains bolted to the bench that was bolted to the floor. He told me to sit back down. I asked him for a cup of water. He told me I couldn't have a cup of water.

Finally, I was on my way to the Austin Department. When he left me at the headquarters, I reached out my hand and shook his, as though to recognize he had done his job. I was searched once again, this time by a different officer, who emptied my pockets into a yellow container. This time they took my cigarettes as well. As I stood there waiting to hear what would happen next, I noticed the mentality of the police officers around me. There had to be at least fifteen or so, most of whom seemed very hostile, walking around cracking loud jokes to each other, as if they needed to fulfill some kind of power trip. Even some of the female officers behaved in this macho manner. I noticed the sign on the wall. It read PEACE OFFICERS. So far what I had experienced since my arrest resembled everything but peace. I kept to myself and stayed polite.

I was directed into a room where I was to wait. For what, I had no clue. I had never been in a situation like this and did not know what would happen next. I sat down on a wooden bench. There were eleven other people in the room. I felt awkwardly out of place. After observing the people in there with me for a while, I picked up one of the four phones on the wall and called my mother. I wondered what time it was and guessed it to be about 2:45 AM. She picked up, and I told her what happened and asked her to do what she could to get me out of there. The door opened. After four other names, mine was called. I told my mom that I had to go and that I would try to call her again.

I had to go with the officer and answer some questions and sign some paperwork. After that, I was asked to take off my shoes and socks and put on a pair of slippers he pulled from the shelves next to me. That moment I knew I was staying longer than I had hoped for. I asked if I could use the bathroom. I could.

Soon after that, me and five others were called, and we were to follow the blue line to the room at the end of the hall. In the room, we were told to take off all our clothes and place them in the bag in front of us. I changed from the clothes I was wearing into a dark blue pajama-like prison suit. Things were looking less bright by the minute. I was given a blanket and directed to follow another blue line upstairs, where another officer took me to my cell.

The bunk bed was already taken. On the floor, in between the bed and the toilet, there was a mattress waiting for me. The guy on top bunk bed was snoring. He must have been in this place for a while. The guy lying on the bottom bunk bed was awake. Like me, unable to sleep. Everything around me was made of steel: the walls, the door, the bunk bed; even the toilet was made of metal. The white fluorescent light behind a metal screen on the ceiling stayed on. All contact with the outside world was cut off. I felt that my very freedom lay in the hands of strange people while all I could do was hope that my mother would get me out of there somehow.

I heard a guard walking toward my cell. *Please let it be for me.* I heard the lock turn and watched the door open. "Hyman," the guard said with a loud voice. I got up and walked out of the cell. "Leave the blanket," he said.

"Am I coming back here?" I asked.

"Eventually."

I followed him downstairs. There was a lawyer there to see me. I felt relieved. He told me I would be out of there in a couple of hours if I signed a paper promising to appear in court. I signed without hesitation.

I felt much better knowing I wasn't going to be there much longer. After I had been back in my steel cage for about thirty minutes, the door opened again. A guard brought in another person. *How many people will they fit in this little room?* I thought. There were now four people in a room no larger than seven by seven feet. The fourth guy laid his mattress half over mine. *Not much longer until I'll be out of this hell.*

Breakfast was served at five thirty in the morning and consisted of an orange, a little carton of milk, and a plastic bag of corn flakes.

At six that morning I was released. I had never appreciated my freedom more than I did that morning. There are still some legal issues to be taken care of, but I am pretty confident it will all work out for the best, and the whole experience has allowed me to learn something I would have never been able to learn in any other way.